WEIGHT LIFTING FOR WOMEN

THE STRONG WOMAN

The Perfect Workout Plan
For Women To Build A
Strong Female Body With
Strength Training

Brisa Singleton

from the Publisher. All additional right reserved.

The information in the following pages is broadly considered to be a truthful and accurate account of facts and as such any inattention, use or misuse of the information in question by the reader will render any resulting actions solely under their purview. There are no scenarios in which the publisher or the original author of this work can be in any fashion deemed liable for any hardship or damages that may befall them after undertaking information described herein.

Additionally, the information in the following pages is intended only for informational purposes and should thus be thought of as universal. As befitting its nature, it is presented without assurance regarding its prolonged validity or interim quality. Trademarks that are mentioned are done without written consent and can in no way be considered an endorsement from the trademark holder.

Table of Contents

PART I

Introduction

The world of strength training is growing increasingly chaotic, and downloading this book is the first step you can take towards getting a little bit more clarity about it. The first step is also always the easiest, which is why the information you find in the following chapters is so important to take to heart as they are not concepts that can be put into action immediately. If you file them away for when they are really needed in the gym, however, then when the time comes to use them, you will be glad you did learn them. What I have discovered after years of strength training, in fact, is that most people think that there is no theoretical aspect behind the exercises they are performing. Instead, knowing it is extremely important to acquiring a better form.

To that end, the following chapters will discuss the primary preparedness principals that you will need to consider if you ever hope to be ready to build up your strength over a period of time. Only by having the right knowledge will you be able to lay out a clear plan to get bigger, leaner and stronger.

In this book, you will learn everything you need to know about strength training and how to take your gains to the next level. The same principles have helped hundreds of other people and me to get the body they desired.

There are plenty of books on this subject on the market. Thanks again for choosing this one! Every effort was made to ensure it is full of as much useful information as possible. Please enjoy!

Chapter 1: How to Choose the Right Number of Repetitions

"How do I choose the number of repetitions and series?"

This is one of the main doubts that assail the neophytes of the gym. I still remember the day I asked my gym instructor about it many years ago. In fact, the first questions that a beginner poses to the instructor in front of a weight machine are typically these: "How many consecutive lifts (or movements) do I have to do with this machines? And for how many times?"

The most precise ones even dare to ask how much time they have to recover from one set to the next one, and so you think you have clarified everything you need to know about a training session at a given weight machine.

The load (i.e., the kg lifted or moved) is generally fixed according to the presumed abilities of the aspiring visitor of the weight room, often without any relation to the first two parameters of repetitions and sets.

There is not a unique answer to these questions since it all depends on the goal. For example, when I first started my training journey, I wanted to get bigger, not stronger. During that period I did a lot of hypertrophy-oriented workouts which worked quite well. When I switched to a more strength-oriented approach, I had to completely rearrange my schedule all over again.

Since the weight training that interests us is not aimed at the practice of bodybuilding—but is framed in the health of those who want to integrate aerobic activities with exercises for the general improvement of strength, elasticity, and flexibility—before defining the number of repetitions and sets, it is necessary to establish the objective to be achieved or what aspect do you want to train for between the following:

- **The resistant force**: the force that the muscle must apply to overcome the fatigue resulting from a prolonged effort.

- **The maximal force**: the maximum force that the muscle can develop with a lifting test (or a limited number of tests). It is also often referred to as a maximal load if referring to a specific exercise in the gym.

- **The fast force:** the maximum force that the muscle can develop to counteract a load in a limited period of time. Referring to time, therefore, more than force we should speak of power which is the ability to develop a force in the unity of time.

- **Muscle hypertrophy**: no reference is made to the type of force that the muscle has to generate, but to its effect on the athlete's body—that is, to maximize the increase in muscle volume. The muscular volume is connected to the developed force, because the greater the cross section of the muscle, the greater the muscle fibers available to make the effort. However, the equation *muscle* *hypertrophy* = *greater muscle strength* is not always true because, in addition to having available muscle fibers, the human body must also know how to recruit, and this is influenced by other factors such as the efficiency of the cardio-respiratory system, the ability coordination, etc. This should make those who seek to maximize muscle hypertrophy think only of achieving the highest possible performance.

In a healthy view of strength training, you can leave out the last point because the search for muscle hypertrophy, typical of bodybuilders, is far from our goals. Therefore, we can identify three types of training, each of which corresponds to a type of strength that you want to train and, consequently, to a pattern of repetitions-number of sets-interval between the different series.

Remember that to define a training plan, the following variables must be defined for each exercise (i.e., for each machine in the gym or exercise with weights):

- Repetition: it is the single gesture of weightlifting or athletic gesture that stresses the muscle or a district of the muscles. Generally, in the gym at each repetition, the muscle or muscles lift or move a weight (load).

- Sets: the consecutive number of repetitions. The set can be slow or fast, or the exercise is done slowly, calmly, or quickly, imposing to adhere to a higher rhythm.

- Recovery: the time between one series and the next.

So, you might find a typical 3-row workout of 12 sets of 25 kg with a three-minute recovery. This is a very standard way to get started and the first style of training that I followed when started out.

Chapter 2: How to Breathe During Exercises

One thing that is often overlooked by many gym enthusiasts is how to perform proper breathing during weight exercises. It is a problem that, sooner or later, most of those who attend gyms propose to their instructor.

Breathing, as we know, is an activity that we do involuntarily, but it is also possible to control it trying to adapt the movement of the muscles (or part of the muscles) involved, such as the diaphragm, the ribcage, the shoulders, abdominals to the rhythm that we want to follow.

Consciously, one can control the inhalation phase and the exhalation phase in their overall duration or even suspend breathing by entering apnoea.

A lot of sports and disciplines (yoga, pilates, etc.), give a lot of importance to breathing, while other oriental disciplines even give it a spiritual value.

Even in the exercises that are performed in the gym, including those with weights, breathing has a considerable importance. Unfortunately, there are not many who have clear ideas about it.

Instructors usually advise to:

- **inhale** in the discharge phase of the action, usually when the weight is being returned to its initial position;

- **exhale** in the loading phase of the exercise or when there is more effort required.

This usually works well, even if the beginner will at first see this as another constraint which will only confuse him. In reality, it requires a good amount of concentration to force yourself to control breathing in this way and therefore forces the athlete to give complete attention to what he is doing. A lot of times, people look around in the gym while doing an exercise, or—worse—talking to someone. This is something that I have never understood: to me, strength training is a way to become the best version of myself, both physically and mentally, and I do not have time to waste. Focusing on breathing is a good way to think exclusively about the exercise you are performing.

The following is a good general rule to follow:

The most important thing to do is not to hold your breath during the loading phase.

Holding your breath in the loading phase is a big mistake, as it is instinctive to hold your breath during the maximum effort required. Instead, the opposite must be done because this practice can also lead to serious consequences, especially if the effort involves muscles of the upper body.

Holding the breath deliberately blocks the glottis, which then leads to a compression of the veins due to an increase in pressure inside the ribcage. As a result of this compression, the veins can also partially occlude (as if they were strangled by one hand) and this considerably slows the return of venous blood to the heart. As a consequence, the arterial pressure rises, reaching even impressive values such as 300 mmHg (usually 120 mmHg at rest). Moreover, as a consequence of the reduced blood supply to the heart, the outgoing blood also slows down and reduces, which decreases the blood and oxygen supply to the peripheral organs. Less blood and oxygen to the brain could result in dizziness, blurred vision, etc. until you eventually faint. These are side effects well-known by opera singers who practice hyperventilation exercises that, in some parts, are performed in apnoea.

Chapter 3: Machines or Free Weights?

The question is interesting, and the purpose of this chapter is to precisely evaluate the advantages and disadvantages of two possible training solutions for muscle strengthening: the use of gym machines or exercise with the aid of free weights.

From a health point of view, it is clear that the question of the title seems reasonable because, unlike in a bodybuilder, muscle strengthening is seen only as a preparatory to a sport or as a general improvement of the body, and therefore it is not said that the use of gym machines is actually the only possible solution for those who want to make a good upgrade without wanting to reach professional levels of a bodybuilding lover. Before analyzing the two solutions in detail, briefly remember that a muscle can perform an effort in two ways of contraction: eccentric or concentric.

In the first case, the muscle develops the force necessary for the exercise when it is stretching, in the second case when it is being shortened.

Weights and machines are not always equivalent in stimulating a muscle in an eccentric and concentric way. For the purpose of training, eccentric work is the most difficult—to the point that it can also induce pain and muscle damage. It is therefore important that, by deciding which exercises to perform (with the machines or with the weights), it is clear (otherwise you can ask the instructor like I did at the beginning of my journey in the gym) which exercises stimulate the muscles more eccentrically, to introduce them gradually into the plan of training avoiding injuries.

Weight Machines

In the gym, there are usually many weight machines. Generally, except for the multi-function stations, each of them trains a specific muscular district or even a single type of muscle. The effort put in place by the muscles during the execution of the exercise must counteract two physical forces: the weight force and the force due to the friction of the weight that it moves (often along ropes or pulleys).

As a general rule of the mechanics involved in the use of weights, during the eccentric contraction, the friction force is subtracted from that of the weight, while during the concentric contraction this force is added.

Free Weights

They are called free-weight exercises because usually the weights are not tied to ropes or pulleys of the machines, but simply gripped or tied to the body (for example with anklets) and carried out only with the aid of weights such as dumbbells and barbells, which are often seen on sale in supermarkets. Surely, compared to a workout with machines, the one with free weights is easier to put in place. Often, it is not even necessary to attend a gym; a small home space equipped with a mat, a bench (if required by the exercises), a mirror (optional, to control the movements) and, of course, the weights is sufficient enough.

Now let's analyze the advantages and disadvantages of the two solutions, taking into consideration some objective parameters that can assume different importance depending on the individual's objectives, the physical state of departure (sedentary, beginner or advanced athlete), and the expectations placed in a training of this type.

- Economic aspect: free weight training is certainly cheaper, because, as mentioned, in most cases it is not necessary to get a gym subscription. It can be a good compromise solution to go to the gym for the time necessary to practice the exercises under the guidance of an experienced instructor, and then, once you are sure to perform the correct movements, buy weights and equip yourself with a training-space inside your home. This is what I did, and I would never go back.

- Versatility: free weights are suitable for multiple exercises and different muscle groups. Think about how many exercises you can do with simple weights to train biceps, triceps, pectorals, etc. In the case of training with weight machines, each machine usually allows a few exercises (if not only one) and this is the practical limit of such a training: you need to choose a gym where there is a sufficient number of machines for the exercises you want to do and where waiting times are not too long. Otherwise, the queues to the machines make the overall workout boring and ineffective.

- Eccentric and concentric training: weight machines usually lesser stress the eccentric work of the muscle (because of the opposing frictional force) unlike the movement of the body which, in returning to the starting position of the exercise, often performs eccentric work of considerable intensity. Moreover, in the exercises with weights, many antagonistic muscles are trained many times, and in general, they also train the balance and proprioceptive, improving body coordination.

- Safety and complexity: from the previous point, we can see that weight machines train specific muscle areas, and it is easier to isolate the muscle or muscle district involved. It is also easier to perform the exercise correctly because the movements are constrained by the machines and are easier to learn. With free weights, it is easier to make mistakes, and generally more antagonistic muscles and the spine are stimulated. In addition, with the weights, it is easier to maintain a constant execution speed. For all these reasons, it is generally said that the exercises with the machines are at a lower risk of injury than those with free weights.

Chapter 4: Putting it all together. How to program a training cycle

Now we come to the crucial point: how do I craft a strength training program? The question is very complex. Each strategy will be based on the condition of the subject, so, logically, when we see a disproportionate lack of strength for a muscle group, it will be logical to intervene in this sense. Let's go step by step. The literature on the subject highlights how, for the purposes of muscular hypertrophy and gains in strength, setting a periodized program is the best solution. Before diving deeper into the topic, it is important to note something. You cannot generalize, there is no way to use a unique approach or way of training a particular component. There are countless cases, solutions. So what can be done is to report different models based on different contexts to give not a guide but a concept—something infinitely more precious (and expendable).

Strategy 1. "Basic" Approach. A first approach that we can use is to set up a multifrequency workout by adopting a daily wavy periodization. So we will have two weekly sessions for each muscle district. In the first session we can train the muscle according to a traditional bodybuilding scheme, then longer TUT, intensity techniques, a range of 8-12 repetitions, eccentric, forced, etc. In the second session, we can train ourselves by adopting a progression of strength. So for example, we will train the chest on a flat bench using possibly another complementary exercise (like crosses, chest fly, etc.). A similar approach is at the base of the PHAT (Power Hypertrophy Adaptive Training) method proposed by

Norton. Unlike this, however, I find it more sensible to use—in training dedicated to strength—real progressions on exercises without being limited to a 5 × 5 standard type of training.

Strategy 2. Deficient Muscles Approach. Similar to the previous one, the only difference is that a workout in this sense will be done on the deficient muscles while the more developed muscles will be trained in mono-frequency. The increase in weekly volume and stimulus variation will bring an advantage in terms of growth (strength and hypertrophy) that will allow you to "catch up" with respect to the rest of the muscles. This approach can be used on deficient muscles both from a hypertrophy point of view and from a force point of view (i.e., the weakest muscles). This last aspect is particularly important as it can be a valid strategy to intervene where a muscle is placed limiting within the synergy of a gesture. The discourse can also be done from the opposite point of view—that is, to hold the strongest or most developed muscle groups to a multifrequency and to mono-frequency to recover asymmetries (aesthetic or functional).

Strategy 3. The transient phase of reduced volume. Another way to insert a strength training within a bodybuilding program is to provide a period with a high load intensity and a reduced volume. In this case, we always speak of wavy periodization. However, the variations will not be done on a daily basis, but weekly. So, for instance, we will put 2-3 up to 6 weeks of strength training with a reduced volume—less dense workouts but with the intensity of high-load and then return, progressively or not, to traditional bodybuilding sessions, or even to a wavy periodization protocol on a daily basis as described above. Basically, it is a matter of setting a transitional phase aimed at two purposes: Varying the stimulus (Ri) and finding the feeling with the motor scheme.

Strategy 4. Periodization within the session. This is also an interesting approach. It is a matter of inserting, within the session, an exercise on which to set up a forced schedule. In this sense, we could then insert the flat bench into a chest session as a first or second exercise. We will choose a program to improve on strength (since we are already able to exercise the right mastery over the exercise) and set the rest of the session as a traditional bodybuilding session. Obviously, the total volume will decrease as part of the session is occupied by dense work—not very voluminous but very intense. I find that such a setting fits well with the daily wavy periodization (strategy 1). Basically, by training a multi-frequency muscle, we will set the strength session using an exercise with its progression and the rest of the session in the traditional bodybuilding style. The diversification of work with respect to the second weekly session will be in the TUT (for example) which, in the latter, will be exasperated (e.g., +50'), while in the session of "strength" it will not be too high (e.g., 30').

Split and choice of exercises

A further aspect on which we must dwell is that relative to the decision, within the session, the target muscle groups and the exercises to be used. One of the characteristics of strength programs is that, in most cases, the various muscle groups are subdivided to work only a few each session. This is logical because the work that is required is always of the same type (anaerobic). Okay, as we have seen, it can work on different adaptive components, but in any case, it is always part of the big family of "boosting" work, the same that, in other sports, is alternated with "technical" work. The question that arises is the following: Should we first set the split and then, based on this, choose the type of exercises in which to work the strength or vice versa? Being a powerlifter myself, I would answer "the second," but from a Bodybuilder perspective I would answer "the first." Since this chapter is about strength training, I would say start from this context and, in particular, from the cases mentioned above. Where we want to set a wavy periodization, for all groups or only for some (strategies 1-2-4), then yes, we will have to start from the split. Based on this we will choose the best exercise on which to progress for the strength. So for example, in a push-day, we will choose the Bench Press for the chest, for a pull-day a Bent Over Row, and for a leg-day a Squat.

Let's do an example: Subject 1, Powerlifter, good management of high loads on the various motor schemes. Deficient groups: Arms, Back. Strong groups: Chest, Quadriceps

Split

Day 1 Push Day

Day 2 Pull Day

Day 3 Leg Day

Day 4 Rest

Day 5 Arms

Day 6 Back

Day 7 Glutes

Logically, we will then insert a progression on the Bent-Over Row on day 2 and work the Back with a traditional strength session on day 6. To evaluate a progression on the ground clearance that would be close to a leg workout (even putting it on day 6), we will have the hamstrings on day 7. But training strength, as we have seen, is not just a matter of periodizing and varying the stimulus, but also a question of functionality to the motor schemes to be performed during the sessions.

So let's take another example. Subject 2: Powerlifter, poor activation of the chest on the bench press, poor feeling on the deadlift. Excellent management of the Squat. Deficient groups: Chest-Back-Arms. The goal, in this case, will be to improve the feeling with easier exercises so we will set the split based on the same.

Split

Day 1 Chest and Shoulders

Day 2 Deadlift day

Day 3 Rest

Day 4 Quadriceps and Arms

Day 5 Rest

Day 6 Chest and Back

Day 7 Arms

Finally, in case we go set up a Strength program as a transitory phase (strategy 3), it will be logical to start from the exercises and, based on these, reason on the split.

PART II

Chapter 1: Setting Yourself Up For Success

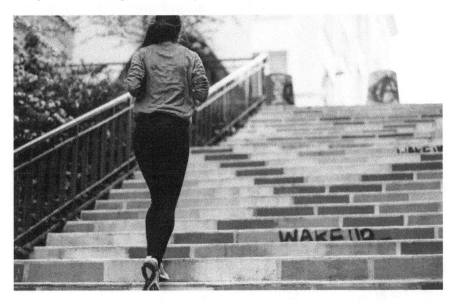

Photo by Ev on Unsplash

How Your Diet Affects Your Results

Exercise and diet are equally important factors to building muscle and losing fat. It is generally touted that diet may even play a larger role in the outcome of your fitness. If you are working out hard and not seeing results, make sure that the things you are eating are unprocessed and have high nutrient values—more specifically, work with a nutritionist to find the macronutrient intake levels that are right for the goal you are trying to reach.

Warm Up Before Working Out

To avoid injury, we should take some time before starting our workout to warm up all of our muscle groups. It is generally accepted that warming up before a workout will lead to better performance results and decrease the chance of injuring yourself. Don't forget to stretch after you're done, too! Warming up and cooling down should take no less than 5 minutes, but no more than 15-20 minutes. We don't want all your time spent prepping for your workout or stretching afterward, but they are important components that ensure your body's continued functionality.

Example Warm Up Workouts:

Complete these exercises for 5-10 minutes

1. Jog, row, or ride a bike at a slow-medium pace
2. Jump rope
3. High knees or butt kicks
4. Walk-out planks
5. Jumping jacks

Important Areas to Stretch:

Areas are followed by examples

1. Arms: arm circles
2. Legs: walking lunges
3. Glutes: glute bridge
4. Calves: wall lean

5. Back: leg pull

When warming up, we want our heart rate to increase, so make sure that while you are completing these exercises, you are adequately exerting yourself. We want our body to be ready for the more intense activity we are about to take part in. An increase in blood flow, an increase in body temperature, and an increase in breathing rate all build slowly through warming up in preparation. If you need to ask yourself if you are working out vigorously enough, a good test to check is to see if you would be able to keep a conversation going with your friend. If you are working out hard enough, you really shouldn't be able to keep a conversation going.

Who These Workouts Are Best-Suited For

Bodyweight Workouts are best-suited for those who cannot afford a gym membership, don't enjoy the gym atmosphere, or for those who feel like they are too large to jump right into fast-paced routines. Memberships can be expensive depending on where you go, and we don't all have enough money to afford one at certain points in our lives. Many people—women, in particular—feel uncomfortable at the gym or are intimidated by the size of the facility and the variety of equipment. Bodyweight Workouts can be modified for someone of any shape and size and can be completed in the privacy of your own home if you are self-conscious by working out in public.

Benefits of Bodyweight Workouts

These workouts allow you to build muscle, gain strength, and increase your stamina by using nothing other than your body. Able to be completed anywhere and with no equipment, Bodyweight Workouts are fast and effective. The Huffington Post contributor Dave Smith lists the numerous benefits of Bodyweight Workouts:

1. They are efficient: "Research suggests high-output, bodyweight-based exercises such as plyometrics yield awesome fitness gains in very short workout durations. Since there's no equipment involved, bodyweight workouts make it easy to transition quickly from one exercise to the next. Shorter rest times mean it's easy to boost heart rate and burn some serious calories quickly."

2. There's something for everyone: "Bodyweight exercises are a great choice because they're easily modified to challenge any fitness level. Adding extra repetitions, performing the exercises faster or super-slow, and perfecting form are a few ways to make even the simplest exercise more challenging. And progress is easy to measure since bodyweight exercises offer endless ways to do a little more in each workout."

3. They can improve core strength: "The 'core' is not just the abs. At least 29 muscles make up our core. Many bodyweight movements can be used to engage all of them. These will improve core strength, resulting in better posture and improved athletic performance."

4. Workouts are convenient: "Ask someone why they don't exercise. Chances are they'll answer they have 'no time' or that it's an 'inconvenience.' These common obstacles are eliminated by bodyweight exercises because they allow anyone to squeeze in workouts any time, anywhere. It can be a stress reliever for those who work at home, or it can be a great hotel room workout for people on the road. With bodyweight workouts, 'no time' becomes no excuse."

5. Workouts can be fun and easily mixed up for variety: "It can be easy to get stuck in a workout rut of bench presses, lat pull-downs, and biceps curls. That's why bodyweight training can be so refreshing: There are countless exercise variations that can spice up any workout routine. Working with a variety of exercises not only relieves potential workout boredom, but it can also help break through exercise plateaus to spark further fitness progress."

6. They can provide quick results: "Bodyweight exercises get results partly because they often involve compound movements. Compound exercises such as push-ups, lunges, and chin-ups have been shown to be extremely effective for strength gains and performance improvements."

Creating a Workout Environment

Since these workouts can be complete at home, making sure you have available space to complete exercises is imperative for success. All you really need is a space large enough to spread out a little bit—let's say for example, to complete 10 lunges in a row. While you do not need any equipment, it may be nice to have a yoga mat if you have hard floors like wood or linoleum.

Some prefer a quiet environment to work out or to use a music player to help them focus during their workout. Do whatever puts you in the zone to complete your routine. The point is to try to minimize the space of distractions so you can put in the work to meet your goals.

Summary and Key Points

- Bodyweight Workouts are easy, fast, and are extremely effective for beginners and more seasoned exercisers!
- You can't expect the most comprehensive results without also ensuring your diet falls in line with the changes you want to see on your body!
- Designate a space to complete your workouts in, whether that be your living room or backyard patio.
- Design your space to allow for workout completion depending on space needs and create motivational vibes in the area for inspiration.

Chapter 2: Types of Bodyweight Workouts

Bodyweight workouts can be focused on targeting a specific group of muscles. This chapter will outline bodyweight exercises that target the following areas: arms, legs, chest, back, butt, and abs.

Photo by Form on Unsplash

We all have what we call 'problem areas,' and strength training can be the best and fastest way to target those areas on our bodies that we want to be more toned. Bodyweight Workouts use our own weight to create resistance so we can work on building up muscle on whichever body parts need our attention. Here are some examples of workouts from the before-named areas:

Focus: Arms

- **Tricep Dips**
  - This move helps build up your pectorals, triceps, forearms, and shoulder muscles. Push your chest out and using your arms, lower your body until your elbows are at 90 degrees. Push back up. Keep your head and chin up during the process.

- **Crab Walk**
  - Get down into a crab position: hands and feet in line with each other and flat on the ground with your chest facing up not down, knees bent, and hips held several inches off the ground. Walk several spaces forward, and then several spaces back.

  - Narrowing your hand placement while completing pushups will engage your core while toning your triceps, pectorals, and shoulders. Start in a pushup position, but instead of your hands lining up with your shoulders, move them in slightly on both sides. Lower your body down, holding yourself up, then push back into the starting position.

Focus: Legs

- **Wall Sit**

o Set your back up against a stable wall until your knees form a 90-degree angle with the wall. Your head, shoulders, and upper back should be lying flat against the wall, with your weight evenly distributed between both feet.

- **Jump Squat**
  o Standing straight up, keep your arms down by your sides. Squat down normally until your upper thighs are as close to parallel with the floor as they can be. Pressing off with your feet, jump straight up into the air, and as you touch down, go back into the squatting position and start again.

- **Lunges**
  o Starting in a standing position, head and chin up, eyes forward, take a step forward with one leg ensuring your knee is above your ankle. You don't want your other knee to touch the ground. Push back up into standing position and step forward with your opposite leg.

Focus: Chest

- **Incline Pushups**
  o This form is a great modification for those who may just be beginning and are struggling to do a basic pushup. Find some kind of incline in your workout area: a desk,

wall, chair, etc. and stand facing the incline with your feet shoulder width apart and feet 1-2 feet back from the wall. Place your hands on either side of the incline and place them slightly wider than your shoulders. Slowly bend the elbows and lower your body toward the incline, pause and push back up—try not to lock your elbows.

- **Traditional Plank**
  - o Start off in a pushup position. Instead of lowering yourself and pushing yourself back up, you intend to hold your body in that position. Do not bend your elbows and make sure your feet are not wider than your shoulders. Hold this pose for 10 seconds to begin, and as you begin to master this exercise, work your way up to 30 seconds, 1 minute, etc.

- **Burpees**
  - o This move combines several moves into one and can be a killer workout for beginners. Standing straight up, bend down in a position with your hands on the floor supporting your body. Kick back both feet until you are in a plank/pushup position. Quickly jump back on your feet and spring up, raising your hands to the sky. After lowering your arms, start again by bending back down.

Focus: Back

- **Reverse Snow Angel**

- Instead of lying on your back like you were about to make a snow angel, flip over and lay face down on the ground. Raise your arms and shoulders off the ground slightly, about two inches, and bring your hands down from your sides up past your head. (If you were standing not laying down you would be raising and lowering your arms in an up and down wing-flapping motion.)

- **Superman**
  - Lie face down on the ground with your toes pointing down under your body. Reach your arms out straight to your sides, and raise both your arms and feet in the air while making sure your torso maintains contact with the ground.

- **Good Mornings aka Hip Hinges**
  - Standing up straight with your hands on your hips and your feet shoulder-width apart, bend forward at your waist until your back is parallel to the ground. Engage your core and bring your torso back up in a straight position. It is important to keep your neck in line with your spine while doing this exercise.

Focus: Butt

- **Fire Hydrants**

- Start in a modified pushup position—the standard pushup position but with knees and hands on the ground instead of feet and hands on the ground. Raise one leg off the ground with your knee bent at a 90-degree angle. This move can also be completed with a straight leg for similar results. If you need inspiration, you want to look like a dog who is just about the use a fire hydrant!

- **Leg Kickbacks**
  - Again, start in a modified pushup position. Try to align your shoulders with your knees. Kick one leg back behind you. Make sure you feel the movement in your hips and glutes, not your lower back. Bring your leg back down and switch sides.

- **Glute Bridges**
  - Lay on the ground, flat on your back with your hands by your sides. Place your feet flat on the floor shoulder-width apart. Use your upper back, upper arms, and core to raise your hips up off the ground toward the sky while keeping your feet and arms on the ground. Slowly lower your hips until they are resting back on the ground.

Focus: Abs

- **Side Planks**

o Lie down on your side on the floor, and place one elbow underneath you so that you are forming a plank on one side. Keeping your elbow underneath your shoulder, push your lower torso up off of the ground so that the only things touching the ground are your right forearm and the side of your right foot or your left forearm and the side of your left foot. Hold the position for ten seconds, release, and then resume the position.

- **Flutter Kicks**
    o Lie on your back on the floor with your arms down by your sides and your heels flat on the ground. Lift your heels about 6 inches off the ground, and quickly kick your legs up and down. It is easier to complete 10 kicks, rest for 20 seconds, then do another 10 kicks because of how short and quick the kicks are.

- **V-Sit Crunch**
    o Lay flat on your back on the ground with your arms laying above your head. Lift up your legs like you are about to attempt a crunch, but bring your arms up toward your legs at the same time, creating a 'V.' Lower your arms and legs back into the starting position lying down.

Summary and Key Points

- There are many more exercises within each focus category. The ones listed in this book are just suggestions to get you started.

- If you are confused about how to complete an exercise, YouTube has an excellent variety of step-by-step videos.

- It's a great idea to track your repetitions (reps), so you know you started being able to do 10 pushups and now doing 25!

Chapter 3: Planning a Workout Routine That Works For You

Bodyweight workouts are perfect because it can be completed with only some space and your body: no gym or equipment required! An even better bonus to these exercises is that they are so simple to do that they are easily combined to reap even more benefits in the same amount of time.

What to Include In Your Plan

Important aspects of a workout routine include duration, frequency, intensity, and consistency. The Mayo Clinic suggests adults get in about 150 minutes of moderate exercise a week, or 75 minutes of vigorous activity and at least 2 days of strength training: "Moderate aerobic exercise includes activities such as brisk walking, swimming, and mowing the lawn. Vigorous aerobic exercise includes activities such as running and aerobic dancing. Strength training can include the use of weight machines, your own body weight, resistance tubing, resistance paddles in the water, or activities such as rock climbing."

To break this down for you, you should look at workouts with moderate intensity for 3 days a week for 50 minutes each, or 5 days a week for 30 minutes each. It's up to you to decide when you want to schedule your workouts throughout the week, but making sure you start your Mondays with a workout is always a great way to set up your week for success!

How to Stay Dedicated When Your Resolve Falters

A LifeHacker article written by Alan Henry has some great tips on how to motivate yourself to start your routine and how to stick with your routine. Without consistency, you will never see or keep results!

1. Stop Making Excuses

   - Don't be too hard on yourself, we all make mistakes and expect too much from ourselves. Know that failures are an expected part of the journey.

   - We all have to start from somewhere—doing something, no matter how small, is better than doing nothing at all!

2. Understand Your Habits

   - "Most people fail in fitness because they never enter a self-sustaining positive feedback loop. To be successful at fitness, it needs to be in the same category of the brain as sleeping, eating, and sex." The key is to find a routine replacement that works for you and gets results for the energy you put into building it into your habits."

   - Starting from zero can cause people to want to give up: "Oftentimes, people are actually lazy because they're out of shape and don't exercise!" It's quite easy for a fit person to tell someone who's having a tough time that they're just lazy, but the reality is that running a mile is much easier for someone who does five every day compared to someone who's been sitting on the couch for most of his life."

3. Find Your "Secret Sauce"

- "Minimizing and oversimplifying the challenge doesn't help, and while hearing what worked for others can help you figure out things to try, it's almost never going to be exactly what works for you. Look for your own combination of tools, tips, techniques, and advice that will support you and your health and fitness goals."

4. Be Engaged and Stick to Your Plan

- "Set the bar low and start small. If you're having trouble with working out every day, start with twice or once a week. Whatever it is, start with something you can *definitely* do effortlessly. This is where suggestions like parking on the far end of the lot and taking the stairs come into play."

- "Whatever you do, make it fun. Whatever you do, enjoy it. Choose something rewarding enough to make you feel good about doing it. If you're having a good time, mistakes feel like learning experiences and challenges to be overcome, not throw-up-your-hands-and-give-up moments."

5. Track Your Victories With Technology

- "Technology can be a huge benefit to help you see your progress in a way that looking in the mirror won't show you. The goal is to keep that track record, whether it's on a calendar, in an app, or on a website, going unbroken as long as possible. Just remember, quantifying your efforts is just a method to get feedback and track your progress. Your tech should be a means to build better habits, not the habit in itself."

Another great way to keep yourself accountable is by enlisting a friend to work out with you. Even if you don't have the same fitness goals or you don't want to be distracted while you are trying to work out, having someone to be accountable to can really push us to meet our goals. Whether that's a text or a phone call on days you know your friend should be working out, that small reminder may be enough to get them going.

Sample 7-day Routine

After deciding how many days and for how long each day you want to work out, the next step is planning what exercises you will complete in each session. It's not generally recommended that you focus on the same muscle groups two days in a row, although every other day is absolutely fine!

Sunday: Arms

15 pushups x3

15 tricep dips x3

15 lay down pushup x3

15 walkouts x3

Monday: Legs

15 jump squats x3

16 X jumps x3

15 lunges x3

24 high knees x3

10 burpees x3

Tuesday: Rest!

Wednesday: Chest

10 second plank x3

15 decline pushups x3

15 mountain climbers x3

15 burpees x3

Thursday: Abs

  15 straight leg sit ups x3

  20 ab bikes x3

  15 straight leg raises x3

  20 side twists

Friday: Rest!

Saturday: Back

  15 bridges x3

  15 back extensions x3

  15 opposite arm/leg raises x3

  15 bridges x3

Try to complete all four workouts on each day as fast as you can while resting for up to 30 seconds between each move. If you want to up the intensity, slowly increase the repetitions—a good interval is an increase of 5. Another way to make the workout more intense is to complete the workout as a circuit. If you complete a day's workouts as a circuit, ignore the "repeat 3 times." Instead, you would complete, for example, 15 straight leg sit-ups, 20 ab bikes, 15 straight leg raises, and 20 side twists. Rest for 30 seconds! Repeat starting with 15 straight leg sit-ups. Try to not rest for more than 30 seconds. If you need to when you're just beginning, that's completely okay! Complete one circuit and begin working on adding additional circuits to your workouts.

If you already have a workout routine that you regularly complete, try adding in certain strength training exercises between your cardio workout. Again, slowly build up your repetitions but starting small.

Summary and Key Points

- Plan your workouts into your day with your planner or calendar system. Start small and build your way up to working out 3, 4, or 5 days a week!

- Switch up the muscle groups you focus on to make sure that you see full body results.

- The recommended workouts are only a very small example of workouts within each category to get you started. Research muscle groups you want to target and incorporate those goals into your workout plan.

Chapter 4: How to Make the Most Out of Your Bodyweight Workouts

As touched on in the last chapter regarding circuit workouts, High-Intensity Interval Training is a great way to target multiple muscle groups in one workout and burn more calories. We will also touch on tools that can be used to track your workouts and your progress, as well as an important aspect of ending your workout that is sometimes forgotten but still important: stretching!

High-Intensity Interval Training

According to Bodybuilding.com, "these different body compositions point to the fact that not all cardio is created equal, which is why it's important to choose a form of cardio that meets your goals. A recent study compared participants who did steady-state cardio for 30 minutes three times a week to those who did 20 minutes of high-intensity interval training (HIIT) three times per week. Both groups showed similar weight loss, but the HIIT group showed a 2 percent loss in body fat while the steady-state group lost only 0.3 percent. The HIIT group also gained nearly two pounds of muscle, while the steady-state group lost almost a pound."

Photo by Autumn Goodman on Unsplash

Progress Can Be Small, But Any Progress is Significant

Tracking your gains is an important part of using body weight workouts. Some people prefer creating their own systems in a notebook or journal, others use electronic devices, and the rest of us prefer to use visual progress indicators.

Writing down when you completed a workout, what exercises you completed, and how many repetitions you completed is a great reminder of your goals and how far you've come on the journey to reach them. Before your next workout, refer back to your last logged workout and see what adjustments you need to make to your workout today to help you be successful.

Technology Can Help Us Keep More Accurate Records

Using a tracking device like a Fitbit watch, hybrid smartwatch, iPhone, or smart shoes, you can track calories burned, distance moved, heart rate, and then have them saved somewhere digitally instead of in a hard copy paper form.

Stretching for Injury Prevention Should Be a Priority

Warming up and then stretching after a workout is an important way to help prevent injuries. Stretch out your arms, legs, back, and any other areas that feel tight.

Key Summary Points

- HIIT workouts are a great way to combine targeting different muscle groups in one workout instead of many.

- Tracking your gains in whichever fashion makes you the most comfortable and that you find the most motivating is highly encouraged!

- Taking 5-15 minutes to stretch after a workout will ease soreness for your workouts in the following days, and will help prevent your muscles from getting   injured.

PART III

Chapter 1: 5 Reasons why most people fail to get bigger

Are you training hard but cannot increase your muscle mass? Read this chapter on the 5 reasons why you are not increasing your muscle mass: you will probably discover that you are making one of these big mistakes. Do not worry, though: understanding the problem is the first step towards solving it.

1. Do you eat enough?

The problem could be easy to solve, do you eat enough? When you embark on a journey into fitness it is can happen to get caught up in exercising and skip on the nutritional aspect. I'm sure you know that 'abs are made in the kitchen'; well, it could not be truer. Eating enough calories (and good ones) is the first step towards getting leaner.

To increase your muscle mass, you have to eat the right amount of the right food, including carbohydrates, proteins, and fats. Your body uses the food you eat to build new muscle tissue after you destroyed the old one in training. In order to do that, it is important to consume enough protein.

Some of the best sources of protein are:

- Chicken

- Fish

- Turkey

- Lean minced meat

- eggs

- meat, broccoli, salmon

Other sources of protein

- Milk flakes

- Greek yogurt

- Quark cheese

- Beans and legumes

- Nuts

A high-protein diet is fundamental to build muscles. Experts and pro bodybuilders have stated, over the years, that consuming 1.2 – 2.0g of protein per kg of weight is a good ratio to keep building lean muscle mass over time. If you are not able to get this amount trough diet alone than food supplements can come handy

2. Do you train hard enough?

If you have been training for a while, but have not made some gains, it could be due to a lack of training. Do you train hard enough? Our body reacts quickly under pressure and if you're not increasing weights over time, then you could run into a stall zone. So do not settle!

Your body is not made to change itself and it is your duty to give it the right stimulus so that it can actually grow. If you want to get faster results, add more intensity to your training.

3. Rest and recovery

Rest is a fundamental aspect when it comes to any fitness routine. Your muscles require rest to grow stronger and that is the reason why so many athletes choose a training routine divided into days. For example, one day they train legs and the day after the arms, making sure that every part of the body receives at least one day of rest (try to train every muscle group at least once a week).

Even sleeping is very important: when we sleep deeply our bodies repair muscle fibres. It is recommended to sleep 8 hours per night, although my advice is to sleep more if you can.

4. Do you drink too much alcohol?

Drinking too much alcohol can destroy muscle growth. Alcohol does not contain valuable nutrients but has many calories, 7 per gram to be precise. As a result, it is easy to "drink your calories" without even thinking about it. If you are on a fitness regimen of any kind, it is advisable to avoid alcohol consumption. However, a drink has never killed anybody, just be reasonable.

5. Are you over-training?

Training with high frequency and intensity activates muscle growth. Therefore, it is fundamental to train different days during the week: 4 days of weight training and 1-2 of aerobic activity is advisable. If you begin a program, complete it! Too many times athletes give up or say that a certain workout does not work "for them" (as if this could be a thing), but the key is constancy. It may take a while to see results, do not give up!

Many bodybuilders, like Arnold, have mentioned the famous 'mind and body connection', so try to keep your attention on the muscle you are training while you do the exercises. It is also a question of 'sensations' and how your muscles contract and expand.

Instead of simply doing the training, focus on the exercise and visualize the growth you are generating.

Chapter 2: 10 Rules to increase your muscle mass

It is always challenging to give the 10 rules of anything. However, when it comes to growing muscles, it is important to have some guidance. This is why we give you 10 rules to increase your lean muscle mass for a more defined body.

- Give space to recovery: it is not true that more is better, especially for the frequency. It is true that you can train only 1 muscle a day and then before you go back to training that muscle should pass 6/8 days, but the organs of "disposal" are always the same and run the risk of overloading. You can make short periods with high frequency, but these must then have periods of supercompensation.

- You should sleep very well: it is not only the quantity (7/9 hours per night) but the quality of sleep. An excellent component of deep sleep, it is the basic element for recovery and growth. Sleep must be mainly nocturnal, it is well known by those who work for shifts that daytime sleep has different qualities.

- Eat often: at least 6 times, breakfast, mid-morning, lunch, afternoon, dinner and after dinner; and in any case, use the rule of about 2.5 hours between one meal and another. If you spend many hours between lunch and dinner, introduce two snacks in the afternoon.

- Eat a balanced diet: with every meal, give space to all the nutrients. Not only proteins and carbohydrates, fats are also great allies, since are hormonal mediators, provide calories and improve recovery.

- Do not train too long: do not spend too much time working on your endurance, since it does more harm than good to muscle's growth.

- Think positive: the mind is a great ally for the optimization of metabolic processes; Positivity helps the hormonal systems to overcome the negativity generated by the inevitable obstacles and setbacks of everyday life. It is essential to define the goals (even in the short term) to go to the gym with clear ideas already, aware that you will have an excellent training session.

- Rely on basic movements: squats, deadlifts, bench, lunges, are the fundamentals; mass is not built by abusing side wings, crosses or arms. Dedicate yourself to these exercises by changing sets, repetitions and recovery times. Then there may be periods in which the complementary serve to unload the joints and give a different kind of intensity.

- Do not just focus on some muscle groups: first, you have to build a solid foundation, do not do like those beginners who already after 6 months want to focus only on one or two muscles.

- Use the right supplements: pay attention, do not abuse them, simply select the main ones; good proteins, BCAAs (branched amino acids) or a pool of amino acids, glutamine, creatine, a support for your joints, HMB. These are already more than enough to support and integrate a diet that must follow the correct guidelines.

- Choose a motivating gym: well-equipped but with what you really need, lots of dumbbells and barbells, benches and maybe 2 racks for the squat. Usually, in these environments, you can also find training partners to share workouts, goals and discussions. Training in a sterile and "losing" environment is certainly not very motivating and does not establish the spirit necessary to achieve the goals.

The points to be developed would still be many but in reality, with the 10 you have read you are already well on your way to get bigger and leaner. Success is built from the basics, especially when you are just starting out.

Chapter 3: How to actually build lean muscles

It is difficult to build muscle mass, but with constancy you can do it; however, if you want to develop it quickly, you can find some compromises, like accept to gain some fat along with muscle mass and stop some other type of training, such as running, so that the body starts to focus on developing muscles. You also need to eat more by using the right strategies and doing those physical activities that allow you to increase your muscles. Here are some of the key steps to build lean muscles for real.

- Start with a basic strength training. Most of the exercises that involve the main muscle groups start with a strength training that activates more joints and that allows you to lift a whole greater weight, such as bench presses for the pectorals, those behind the head for the deltoids, the rower with a barbell for the back and the squats for the legs. They are all exercises that allow you to lift heavier weights while still remaining active and keeping enough energy to better stimulate muscle growth.

- Engaged thoroughly. The key to developing muscle mass is to do high intensity exercises; with a light exercise, even if protracted in time, the muscles almost never find the right conditions for decomposition and then rebuild. Schedule sessions for 30-45 minutes 3-4 times a week (every other day); it may seem like an easily manageable schedule but remember that during each session you have to engage as intensely as possible. Initially, the muscles may be sore, but over time the routine will become easier.

- During each training session, only lift the weights that you are able to support by assuming the correct posture. Test your limits to find the right ballast you can lift, doing different repetitions with different dumbbells. You should be able to do 3-4 sets of 8-12 repetitions without feeling the need to put them on the ground; if you are not able, reduce the weights. In general, 6-12 repetitions stimulate the growth of the volume of the muscles, while fewer repetitions favour the increase of the strength at the expense of the size of the same. If you can do 10 or more repetitions without experiencing a burning sensation, you can increase the weight; remember that you do not increase muscle mass until you challenge yourself to the limit.

- Lift weights explosively. Raise the handlebars quickly but lower them slowly.

- Keep the correct posture. To develop a precise technique, you have to do each repetition in the right way; beginners must commit to doing only the repetitions that they are able to perform based on the level of resistance. Find your rhythm for each exercise; you do not have to reach muscle failure when you're at the beginning. You should be able to complete the whole movement without getting to bend down or change position; if you cannot, switch to less heavy dumbbells. In most cases, it starts with the arms or legs extended. During the first sets, you should work with a personal trainer who will teach you the correct posture of the various exercises before continuing alone.

- Toggle the muscle groups. You do not have to keep the same group moving at every set, otherwise, you may get to damage your muscles, so be sure to alternate, so every time you train you can work intensely for an hour on a different muscle group. If you do physical activity three times a week, try doing the exercises as follows:

First session: do exercises for the chest, triceps and biceps;

Second session: concentrate on the legs;

Third session: do abs and chest

- Be careful not to reach a stall level. If you always do the same exercise repeatedly, you cannot get improvements; you have to increase the weight of the barbell and when you reach a plateau even with this, change exercise. Be aware of progress and see if your muscles do not seem to change, because it may be a sign that you need to make changes in your physical activity routine.

- Rest between one workout and another. For those who have a rapid metabolism, the rest period is almost as important as the exercise itself. The body needs time to regenerate muscle mass without burning too many calories by doing other activities. Running and other cardio exercises can effectively prevent muscle growth; then take a break between the different sessions. Sleep well at night, so that you feel regenerated for the next session.

- Create a mind/muscle connection. Some research has found that it can optimize results in the gym. Instead of focusing on your day or the girl next to you, committed to developing a muscle-oriented mindset that helps you achieve your goals. Here's how:

Every time you complete a repetition, visualize the muscle growth you wish to achieve.

If you are lifting with one hand, place the other on the muscle you wish to develop; in this way, you should perceive exactly which muscle fibres are working and you can stay focused on the effort.

Remember that the amount of weight on the bar is not as important as you may think, but it is the effect that weight has on the muscle that allows you to get the volume and strength you are looking for; this process is closely related to the mentality and the goal of your concentration.

- Eat whole foods rich in calories. You should get the calories from nutritious whole foods, so you have the right energy to quickly accumulate muscle mass. Those rich in sugar, white flour, trans fats and added flavours contain many calories but few nutrients and increase the fat instead of developing the muscle. If you want to develop the muscles and their definition, you have to opt for a wide variety of whole foods that are part of all the food groups.

- Eat protein rich in calories, like steak and roast beef, roast chicken (with skin and dark meat), salmon, eggs and pork; proteins are essential when you want to increase muscle mass. Avoid bacon, sausages and other sausages, because they contain additives that are not suitable if you eat it in large quantities.

- Consume lots of fruit and vegetables of all kinds; these foods provide the essential fiber and nutrients, as well as keeping you well hydrated.

- Do not neglect whole grains, such as oatmeal, whole wheat, buckwheat and quinoa; avoid white bread, biscuits, muffins, pancakes, waffles and other similar foods.

- Add legumes and nuts, such as black beans, Pinto, Lima, walnuts, pecans, peanuts and almonds to your diet.

- Eat more than you think you need. Eat when you're hungry and stop when you feel satisfied? This may seem completely normal, but when you're trying to gain muscle mass quickly, you have to eat more than usual. Add another portion to each meal or even more if you can handle it; the body needs the energy to develop the muscles: it is a simple concept.

To this end, a good breakfast includes a cup of oatmeal, four eggs, two or more slices of grilled ham, an apple, an orange and a banana.

For lunch, you can eat a wholemeal sandwich with chicken, several handfuls of dried fruit, two avocados and a large salad of cabbage and tomatoes.

For dinner, you can consider a large steak or some other source of protein, potatoes, vegetables and double the portions of each dish.

- Eat at least five meals a day. You must not wait to be hungry before eating again; you have to constantly replenish your body when you are trying to develop muscle mass. It will not be this way forever, so take advantage and enjoy the moment! Eat two more meals in addition to the traditional three (breakfast, lunch and dinner).

- Take supplements, but do not solely on them. You do not have to think that protein shakes do all the work for you; for your purpose, you need to get the most calories from high-calorie whole foods; Having said that, you can definitely speed up the process by taking certain supplements that have not proven to be harmful to the body.

Creatine is a protein supplement that can increase muscle; usually, it is sold as a powder that is dissolved in water and drunk a few times a day.

Protein shakes are fine when you cannot get enough calories through normal meals.

- Keep yourself hydrated. Training hard to gain muscle mass can quickly dehydrate you. To cope with this risk, always carry a bottle of water with you wherever you go and drink whenever you are thirsty; in theory, you should drink about 3 litres of fluids a day, but you should drink more, especially before and after training.

Avoid sugary or carbonated drinks, because they do not help your overall fitness and may even take you back when you do strength exercises.

Alcohol is also harmful for your purpose: it dehydrates and leaves a feeling of exhaustion.

- Try to get to know your body better. Do you know which foods are effective for you and which are not? During this phase of change, pay attention to what happens to your muscles. Each person is different and the food that is not suitable for one person can instead be very useful for another; if you do not notice improvements within a week, make changes and try something else the following week.

- Sleep more than what you think you should. Sleep is essential to allow muscles to develop; try to sleep at least seven hours a night, although the ideal would be 8-9 hours.

- Focus only on strength training. You may like to do cardio exercises (sports like running and so on), but these activities require a further effort of the body (muscles and joints) and consume the energy you need to build muscle mass. In general, cardio activities should be included in an exercise routine for general health and well-being, but if you are currently struggling to increase muscle volume quickly, you need to focus on this for a few months, so you can reach your goal.

Chapter 4: Tips to keep making gains

- Always ask a friend for help when doing the most difficult lifting exercises, such as bench press; these are high risk movements and it is always important to have some support to be able to do more repetitions.

- Keep motivation high. Find a friend who's training with you, sign up for a weightlifting fan forum or keep a diary to monitor progress; whatever you choose, the important thing is that you inspire yourself.

- If you currently do not have dumbbells and you've never done weight lifting so far, start with push-ups and chin-ups, which are quite challenging for a beginner.

- Make the push-ups easier: start from the normal position of the push-ups and lower the body very slowly; go down as far as possible without touching the floor with your chest and abs. Later, relieved after resting your knees on the ground and start again. This is an excellent solution when you are not yet strong enough to be able to do traditional push-ups.

- Make sure you stay focused. Take breaks only when you need them and not when you feel tired; it is only in this way that you can develop psychological endurance.

Chapter 5: Example of a training schedule

The frequency of this hypothetical schedule for mass training, provides 4 days of training per week, with about 10-12 repetitions per exercise.

The mass program is a middle ground between heavy weights / high intensity training and volume/pump training. You work on strength, hypertrophy, rotating muscle definition and progression, accustoming the body to weight and intensity of work with a growing load plan, which reaches your ideal combination for mass growth.

It is essential, in fact, to know your body and your own ceilings, to prepare and act upon a successful program.

Weekly training schedule (Monday - Friday)

Chest and abs

Legs

Rest

Shoulders - triceps

Back - biceps

Daily mass gym program

1st day - chest and abs

crossed exercises with dumbbells - flat bench

distances with barbell - flat bench

multipower inclined (or with dumbbells)

cross exercises with cables

crunches (3 sets - 15 repetitions)

abs with elbows in support and knees on the chest (3 sets - 15 repetitions)

2nd Day - legs

45-degree press

squat with barbell

standing calf (3 sets - 15 repetitions)

seated calf (3 sets - 15 repetitions)

leg extension

leg curl

3rd Day - shoulders and deltoids

slow forward exercise with barbell - seated

pull at the bottom with a barbell

lateral raises with dumbbells

push down

French press around the neck with a barbell

bench presses

4th Day - back

pull ups

pullover

pulley

deadlift

curl with dumbbells

curl reverse socket with a barbell

Recovery between the series should be carried out for about 1 minute and a half (1 '30).

The first month these exercises should be performed with at least 3 sets and about 10-12 repetitions, with non-high loads. In case you are not trained enough, you can think of sets of 12-10-8 repetitions, where you start with 12 and perform 8 repetitions in the third set.

The second month you can go up to 4 sets with 10 repetitions or 12 if the body keeps up with the pace. It will not be easy to get to the twelfth repetition without fatigue and, in this case, you can also think about dropping with weights and get to 12 repetitions with lighter loads.

The third month you have to keep the pace but without progressing too much, with the initials 3 sets of 12 repetitions per exercise.

PART IV

Chapter One: Muscle Mass

You have probably heard by now of the many benefits of having more of your body being composed of muscle mass. And yet, I'd venture to guess you still don't know the half of it!

If you're a woman, thirty percent of your body is made up of muscle mass; for men, it's around forty. The bottom line is, we all want more muscle! Muscle gives us that long and lean appearance—with nicely shaped muscles. Muscular people are viewed as healthy people. Obviously, they are also stronger. Too much fat can lead to all kinds of health problems, not to mention all the clothes you have that you can't wear!

There are many, many reasons to desire to build more muscle, but I'll give you the one that is at the top of the list for me: muscle burns fat. That's right! Muscle burns fat not only when you're in the gym or somewhere else, hitting the weights, or doing body resistance training, it does so when you're at rest. That is correct. Muscle eats away at fat while you're lolling on the sofa watching that Sunday afternoon football game.

This is why we love muscle!

Many folks don't do weight training because they think they have to head to the gym. It's a very common myth that it's necessary to use weights in order to add muscle. But it's just that—a myth. You also don't have to purchase a room full of expensive weights, gadgets and other equipment to use to build muscle at home.

I'm going to let you in on a little secret. You can build muscle using just...you. It is true. You can use your own body's resistance against itself to burn fat and build muscle. It's awesome! This way, there are no excuses. You don't have to pay a gym membership, drive yourself there, or even leave the comfort of your own home.

I'm going to give you nine different muscle-building, fat-burning workouts, and we're going to talk—just a little—about a few things you can do in the area of diet. Yes, diet. Not "diet" as in a bad word—like "I feel miserable after eating badly for the last two weeks and I need to go on a diet." Not that sort of talk. We'll simply touch on some of the foods you should be eating and some of the food you shouldn't be if you're genuinely interested in losing some weight.

Before we get into the exercises, let's cover some basics.

How Muscle is Built

Simply put in laymen's terms, when you work out, you essentially damage your muscles. Muscle tissue is broken down. When this process happens, your body gets busy repairing and replacing these damaged tissues. To get just a little technical during this process, the body has a process on the cellular level in which it repairs or replaces the damaged muscle fibers. It fuses these fibers together to form new myofibrils (muscle protein strands). Repaired myofibrils are larger in thickness and are greater in number, thus causing muscle hypertrophy (growth). This process doesn't happen when you are lifting weights, though. It happens afterward when the body is at rest. That's why rest is absolutely a key component to muscle growth. The hard work is only half the process. But fortunately the rest—pun intended—is easy.

Chapter Two: The Upper Body

"Can we please have a moment of silence for all those stuck in traffic on the way to the gym?" —Anonymous

These aren't always the easiest exercises to do—well, actually, exercising isn't exactly easy anyway, so scratch that. The great thing about upper body work is that this is where you will begin to see results first. So, for that reason, doing upper body work can be incredibly rewarding.

1. The Classic Push-Up

Push-ups are super easy, super basic and have been around forever. The reason they've been around forever is that they're also super effective. The key is to perform them correctly. If you don't, they become wasted effort.

The proper way to do push-ups

Get on the ground, belly down. Place your palms on the floor a shoulder width apart or slightly more. Keep your body straight as you push yourself up by extending your arms. Repeat. Make sure that your arms are lifting your body weight, not the muscles on the lower half of your body. Imagine there is a plank of wood on your back starting from your head to your feet. Make sure that your body is as straight as that plank in order to maintain correct body alignment.

How many push-ups?

That depends on the kind of shape you are in when you start. When you begin to do the push-ups, do they feel easy to you? Make sure you are performing the move deliberately—not going too fast that you're using momentum. The first time you try, do as many as you can while still keeping perfect form. Afterward, for your regular sets, do two-thirds that many. So, if you did fifteen but were tired by then and beginning to lose form, use ten as a target for your sets in the beginning.

As you get stronger, make the number higher. You want to continue to be challenged. Some people do as many as one-hundred push-ups per day. Perhaps that's something you can aim for. For the average beginner, three sets of ten are reasonable.

2. Chair-Dips

This is another upper-body exercise that, while in actuality, you're using your body-weight, you'll still need a chair or a bench or something similar. When I'm out running, there's a square cement planter that has an edge to it, and it works perfectly.

Dips further work the rhomboid muscles in your back and synchronize with push-ups on working your triceps.

- Get a chair/bench or another object capable of supporting your body weight and of a similar height, as explained above. Stand with your back to it. Make sure that the object is sturdy enough to support your entire body weight. Lower yourself and place your palms on the front edge of the bench, fingers pointing forward. Tuck in your elbows to your sides. Maintain this position and walk just your feet slowly in front of you. Your body weight should be resting on your arms now. Deliberately bend your arms and lower yourself. Do this until the floor is parallel to your upper arms. If you're doing it right, you'll feel it in your back and also in your triceps. Simply hold for about a second and return to the starting position.

Do three sets. Determine the number of repetitions per set the exact same way as you did for the push-ups.

3. Diamond Push-Ups

Oh, chicken wings—and not the kind you eat. "Chicken wing" is a common term used to refer to the fat on the back of a person's upper arm as it kind of tends to sag, resulting in an unattractive "flapping in the wind" sort of scenario when you wave your arms. Nobody has time for this, people! Not when there are exercises that will blast those wings if you simply stay consistent. Almost everyone wants tight, toned arms. It's a sexy look, and it's youthful! Tight triceps can actually defy a woman's age. So don't skimp on the upper body exercises. I'm giving you three here, and all of them work your triceps, but the Diamond Push-Up works it the most of all so if you're only worried about triceps and nothing else, do this one.

- Start in the push-up position, yet instead of having your hands out to the sides, place them in front of you and put them together to create a diamond shape.
- Raise yourself until your legs are straight then lower yourself until you are two inches above the ground. You will feel the burn in those triceps. Embrace the burn! The burn means the move is working.

Choose your number of reps in the same manner with all of the upper body   exercises.

81

Chapter Three: The Core

You must not ignore the importance of core work when it comes to resistance training. Your core muscles are the ones that essentially holds everything else together.

There's a very good chance that, no matter what you're doing, you're using your core. Having a weak core takes the power away from all the rest of your muscles. Your core muscles are also responsible for your balance and stability, which is huge. Your core is not one muscle; it's a complicated interconnected series of muscles which effectively include all of them except your arms and your legs. So, I reiterate. Working your core needs to be an incredibly important part of your exercise routine.

Think about your abs. Everybody seems to be concerned with their abdominal muscles. Many people want those six-pack muscles to show. Some just want to button their favorite jeans without lying on the bed.

There's a common misconception (still) that fat can be "spot-burned." This is simply not true. The general consensus is that fat leaves the body the same way it came on—gradually and kind of all over. Don't get me wrong on this; genetics do play a role in how our bodies store fat. Some people can be perfectly proportioned pretty much everywhere on their bodies and yet have large, unattractive bellies. Those people are still more the exception than the rule.

So, the bottom line is that you cannot target fat-burning. If you really want the fat to leave your body, there are three central areas that will require your attention: diet, cardio, and resistance training. Here we are focusing on the third, and a little later I'm going to give a quick overall snapshot of the importance of combining all three.

I'm going to give you three exercises for your core. This first one, known as a Plank, could actually be used as the only core exercise you do. It is that effective and, especially considering the other exercises you'll be doing with, will touch all the muscles in your core.

Now, remember what we said about abs and fat? Here's something many people simply don't realize. Underneath however much fat we happen to be carrying on our abdominal muscles, we all have a "six-pack." Those are muscles in each of our bodies. What people are trying to do when they say they're going for six-pack abs is burn the layers of fat that cover those muscles. As I said, and much to the sadness of myself and many others, you can't target that weight.

Additionally, I'm not going to include any kind of "sit-ups" in upper body work. They've been proven to not be as effective as other exercises that work the core muscles. Also, I personally think that unless your form is always perfect with a sit-up, you may be putting certain back muscles at risk.

4. Plank

This one is tough, but like I said, with this one exercise and all the many variations you can do with it, you can get those core muscles strong in no time.

- Start with the initial push-up position. Bend your elbows to a right angle. Let your weight rest on your forearms. You might want to get a mat or something soft to use as padding between your arms and the floor. Make sure you have a timer too. The elbows need to be beneath your shoulders directly. Your body should be forming a straight line from head to heels—like a plank. Hold this position for as long as you can without injuring yourself.

Your goal should eventually be to hold it for two minutes. I said eventually for a good reason. Planks are tough. I mean, for a lot of people, a ten-second plank and they're toast. Because so many muscles are used to hold this position, if those muscles aren't strong, it simply can't happen for very long. That's also why planks are such a good indicator of how far you've come. If, when you start it takes all you have to hold a thirty-second plank, I would venture to guess that after a religiously followed routine, within eight weeks you will have worked up to the full two minutes.

Planks are great because there are many variations of them, as well. As you get stronger, try this:

- While in plank position, lift one of your legs as high as you can and hold it there for a count of thirty. Repeat on the other side.
- You can even do a side plank. Lay down on your side with your head propped on your elbow, raise your body in that position and hold it. To increase difficulty with this one, once you are in the up position, try raising your top leg and holding it in that position.

Planks can be thought of as a "Super Move." They literally work all of your muscles. In fact, if one really wanted to, one could do planks only as their resistance training (planks in all their variations, which are many) and achieve the results they're looking for.

5. Reverse Crunch

Okay, so I realize I just got done telling you that sit-ups, which are essentially crunches, are not good for the back muscles. In fact, one physician has said that he has seen no other cause of back injury with the highest rate as traditional crunches.

However, the reverse crunch, despite its name, does not carry the same risks and is excellent at targeting your abdominal muscles.

Here's how to do it:

- Lie down on the floor and fully extend your arms and legs to the sides. Put your palms on the floor. Your arms should actually stay in one place as you perform the entire exercise.
- This is the position you will start from: your legs will be pulled up which will make your thighs form a right angle with the floor. You will want your feet together and also parallel to the floor.
- Move your legs towards your torso. At the same time, roll your pelvis backward. Raise your hips above the floor. The goal is to have your knees touching your chest.
- Hold this position for around a second, then lower back to the starting position.

Again, depending on your ability when you start, gauge the number of reps and sets by how they feel to your body and how hard it is for you to do them at first. Just make sure not to overestimate yourself too much. Muscle soreness from overdoing it is no fun!

6. Mountain Climber

Get into the top of the push-up position. This is the starting position.

- Keeping your back in a straight line, bring your right knee toward your chest. Quickly bring it back to the starting position. Do the same for the left knee. Repeat but speed up the movement, alternating legs quickly as if you were running in place with your hands on the ground.

As far as how many sets, this move isn't exactly structured that way so use seconds to guide you. Try the move until you are really struggling to continue (you'll likely be out of breath) then use two-thirds of those seconds, call it a set, and do three.

Chapter Four: The Lower Body

Working out your lower body is not to be taken lightly or skimped on when doing resistance training. One particular reason for this is because your lower body contains the largest muscle in your entire body: the gluteus maximus.

Not only do most of us like to work out this muscle because it makes us "look" better, it's also a powerhouse. This muscle, along with other gluteal muscles, is one of the great stabilizers of the human body. Keeping these muscles strong can minimize aches and pains in your lower back and hips. The muscles also give you the power you need to do simple things like walk, run, and climb.

So, whenever lower body resistance training is discussed, there are two moves that are practically givens. No, it's not because they're both somewhat torturous—it's because they are effective!

When you're doing your workout, never forget the old adage, "Pain is temporary...(fill in the blank)." Usually, people say, "pain is temporary, quitting lasts forever."

That doesn't exactly apply here, but the point is that if you aren't going to be able to tolerate a little bit of pain, you aren't going to get the same results. Workouts can hurt. Muscles burn. Sometimes by the end of a good workout, you feel like you're about to croak. As far as I'm concerned, those are the very best kind! It means you've really kicked some gluteal maximuses and made some progress for the day. You have to maintain a good attitude if you're going to embark on this journey. Results don't happen overnight, but relatively you will start to see them very quickly (although, in general people who are close to you will notice before you do.) However, nothing is more satisfying than when you do look in the mirror and see results that can't be denied, or when you put on a pair of jeans that has been an eternity since they were last wore and they button easily. It's a powerful feeling.

So, here they come, the not-always-fun but ever-so-productive lower body movements.

7. The Lunge

If you've ever done them, you're probably feeling the burn simply at the thought! When executed correctly, these babies do burn, but they are incredibly effective.

Lunges produce fast results. You will notice that your legs and derriere are more toned and attractive looking. You will feel that you're stronger and you'll notice the difference when you do cardio—assuming you do, of course.

Lunges do not require weights, although weights can be added later on to increase the difficulty as you get into better shape.

Form in lunges is very important. The same is true with all of these exercises. If you're going to put in the effort, you may as well make sure you're doing it right in order to maximize your results.

Following is how to execute a perfect lunge:

- Stand upright and keep your body straight. Pull your shoulders back and relax your chin. Keep your chin pointed forward, don't look down. Make sure the muscles in your core are tight and engaged.

- If it helps you with balance, you can use something you have on hand, like, say, a broom. Hold it crossways in front of you and let it lightly rest on your shoulders.

- Pick a leg. Step forward using that leg. Lower your hips until both your knees are forming a right angle. Make sure that your lowered knee isn't touching the floor and that your forward knee is directly above your angle and not too far forward. Make sure that your weight is in your heels as you push yourself back up to the starting position.

- When you do push back up to the starting position, really place extra emphasis on engaging your gluteus maximus. Deliberately use the strength in that muscle to push yourself upright.

Now. Repeat. How many times? I recommend starting with three sets of ten perfectly executed lunges. If you don't feel "the burn" add a couple, or go ahead and use a barbell if you have one and put some weight on it. You can even do lunges in reverse, to vary things up.

8. Squat

Ah, the squat. If you haven't done them, you've probably heard of them if you have any friends at all who work out. Like lunges, they are simple, easy to execute, and incredibly effective at increasing muscle mask and making you stronger.

Also, like lunges, there are quite a few variations to squats that you can use as you get more fit. For now, of course, we'll focus on the simple squat. Again, form is super important.

- Stand with your feet at least shoulder-width apart. If you feel more comfortable, it's okay to place your feet a bit wider apart. As you stand, you should focus on having your weight on your heels. Extend your arms straight out. The first thing you'll do is thrust your hips back slightly as though you are about to take a seat. Then, lower yourself down like that as if you are actually about to sit down. You'll want to go as low as you can. The goal is to make your knees bent so that your legs are parallel to the floor, again almost if you were sitting in a chair. Control your knees so they don't move forward over your feet.

- The next step is simply to stand up, and when you are coming upright, squeeze your glutes at the top of the movement. So, essentially, squats are like sitting in an invisible chair, then standing up using your glutes to propel you. Very easy but super effective!

9. The Bridge

The bridge is another great one for strengthening your glutes and legs. Remember, before you even see the results of these exercises, you'll be stronger for doing them. And, if you eat right and take in enough protein (building blocks for muscle) you will increase the size of your muscle and consequently burn fat. So when you're doing these not-so-fun-at-the-time moves, keep that in mind!

- Here's how to do a bridge: Lie on the floor, flat as a pancake. Place your hands on your sides and bend your knees. Your feet should be about shoulder-width apart. Lift your hips off the floor, using your heels to push. Keep your back straight while doing this! Hold the position for a second and squeeze those glutes.

- Slowly lower back to the position you started from.

For the number of reps, use the method we discussed previously. The first time you try the exercise, go until you really feel the burn—until it's very tough to continue or until you would not be able to. However many reps that is (say it's fifteen) subtract one-third of that number and start from there.

For variety, this exercise can be performed with one leg at a time.

Chapter Five: Putting it all Together

People have different preferences in how they like to work out. To see good results from strength training, you need to work each muscle group no less than two times per week. Three times is fine and you may see faster results that way. Depending on what you want to accomplish, generally, three times is enough.

The idea is to give each muscle group a rest day in between your workouts. So people go about the entire construct differently. Some like to work their entire body in one session, then rest for a day or two and do it again, up to three times a week.

Others prefer to break the muscle group workouts up. Legs one day, arms the next, core the next, like that.

In my opinion and in consideration of the research I've done, any of the above-mentioned ways to go about it will be just as effective as another. Of course, the most important component is that it gets done.

I'd like to take a moment at the time to talk about cardiovascular workouts. I know, I know, boo, hiss. A lot of people really aren't that big on cardio. However, there's a lot to be said for a good cardio sweat session. For one thing, cardiovascular exercise improves the health of our heart and lungs. That alone should be reason enough to work some in. Also, this type of exercise, depending on the type you choose, can burn an awful lot of calories. Remember, any calories burned will contribute to that sleek, muscular look. For the muscles to come out, the fat has to come off.

Cardiovascular exercise has also been proven to affect our moods in a positive way (the same can be said for weight training.)

The best, most well-rounded exercise plans include a mixture of both. Supposing you hate cardio, you will do yourself no harm by keeping it to a minimum. The general recommendation right now is to get thirty minutes of cardio on "most" days of the week.

Given that, as an example, you could do your weights on Monday, cardio Tuesday, weights Wednesday, Cardio Thursday, weights Friday and guess what? Take the weekend off!

This is just one example of how this can all be done. You can be as creative as you want to be or as you need to be to get around a work schedule.

You could do, for instance, cardio in the morning and resistance training at night. You could work in all or part of your resistance training during your lunch hour at work.

There are no limits to the options available, so that simply means *no excuses*.

No equipment or anything fancy is required for the cardio portion either. Walking is cardio. Just walk fast enough to get your heart rate up, break a sweat and breathe a little heavy. Increase intensity as your fitness level improves.

Here's a sample plan, if you need one. I'm going to use ten reps as a standard while performing the strength training for the sake of simplicity.

Monday Morning Before Work:

Three sets of ten of each of the following:

- Push-ups
- Chair-Dips
- Diamond Push-ups

Honestly, this should take you no more than ten minutes.

Monday Lunch:

- Walk for thirty minutes

Monday Evening:

Perform three sets of the following:

- Squats
- Lunges
- Bridges
- Planks
- Mountain Climber
- Reverse Crunch

Starting out, repeat this same routine on Wednesdays and Fridays. Try this for a few weeks (or another plan of your own design) and see how it works with your schedule.

On the days that you don't walk for thirty-minutes on your lunch, per your official "schedule," do it anyway. If not that, jump on the trampoline with your little ones at night for half an hour. Ride your bike. Swim. Ski if you live near snow and/or if it's wintertime. Snow Show. Or...head to the gym. Do the elliptical or the stair-climber for half of an hour. It's really not hard to get in the minimum amount of cardio and depending on your goals, and who says you have to stop with the minimum?

If you stick to this program, you're going to see some results and you'll see them pretty quickly.

Here's another tip: throw away your scale. Okay, well you don't have to throw it away. I just don't recommend weighing yourself all the time. It could discourage you in fact, for the simple reason that muscle actually does weigh more than fat. You might gain in the beginning, and no one wants to start a workout program only to see the numbers on the scale go up. No way! Instead of worrying about the scale, judge your progress by—most importantly—how you feel, and as for changes in your body, you can always take some initial measurements and then re-measure once a week. What has always worked best for me is simply to gauge how my clothes fit. That's the biggest tell of all. I have a pair of jean shorts I'm wearing right now. A couple of months ago I couldn't get them to even think about zipping! That's the only kind of progress I need. To me, numbers on the scale don't mean a whole lot.

Chapter Six: On Your Diet

It wouldn't be right to talk about gaining muscle and losing fat without talking a bit about diet.

I'm not going to go overboard but there are a few things I'd like to touch on.

First off, as I previously spoke about at the end of chapter four—the scale—I forgot to mention another reason I don't care to use them. Most of them have a tendency to fluctuate as much as five pounds in less than twenty-four hours. In other words, if I'm going by the scale, I often will have "gained" five pounds from when I got up to when it's time for bed.

Not cool.

Not possible, either. Our bodies are made up of an estimated sixty-five percent water. It is normal for the amount of water in our bodies to fluctuate all the time. Losing water weight does not equate to losing fat. However, while we are trying to lose weight, and while we're working out, it is especially important to keep our bodies hydrated.

There are as many theories on the web as you could click on about how much water to drink, but for questions like these, I like to refer to the Mayo Clinic website, because I know that the information they put out there has been thoroughly researched. What follows is their advice on water intake:

Every single day, you lose water by breathing, sweating, urinating, and pooping. To function properly, your body's water must be replenished through the consumption of food and beverages.

The average healthy man who lives in a temperate climate needs 15.5 cups or 3.7 liters of fluids every day, and the average healthy woman living in the same place needs 11.5 cups or 2.7 liters every day.

This is about what I do for myself in a normal day and it seems to work. Regardless, don't skimp on the water.

There's another important factor when it comes to building muscle and that is protein. If you are serious about adding some muscle mass, you're going to need to eat your protein. That doesn't mean it has to be meat; there are plenty of non-meat options for protein intake. Of course, if you are a vegetarian you already know that.

Another little tip: your body needs fat to lose fat. Sounds strange, doesn't it? But if your body is starved of nutrients, it will begin to hold on to everything it has instinctually, and as a result, you won't see any weight loss.

There are a million types of "diets" out there, and this is not a book about diets so I'm not going to delve into them. If I were going to say anything at all about your diet (and don't get me wrong, your diet IS important,) I would say two words: eat clean.

What does that mean? Since clean is the opposite of dirty, in this case, think dirty equals "processed."

Do your body a giant favor and stay away from processed foods! Eat foods that are as "close" to the earth as you can.

- Lean proteins (including fish and non-meat proteins)
- Tons—and I do really mean tons—of vegetables
- Lean fat (avocado, almonds, coconut oil)
- Dairy (full-fat; eat sparingly)
- Fruits (sparingly)

It's that simple. No "TV Dinners." No boxes of macaroni and cheese, please. Nothing that has a "bunch" of ingredients, many of which you aren't even familiar with. Those are bad. Leave them in the store.

If you have a sweet tooth, indulge it, but rarely, and even a sweet tooth can be indulged in a healthy manner. There's nothing wrong with eating some strawberries topped with full fat whipped cream. Yummy!

Well, there you have it. You really are set. Everything is explained and condensed for you.

Start your weight training and your cardio, eat clean, drink your water and reap the rewards.

Go get 'em!

PART V

Chapter 1: Keto Basics

Benefits of Increased Metabolism

One of the best ways to learn the meaning of a scientific term is to break it down to its roots. When we break down ketogenic, we see it is comprised of two words: keto and genic. Ketones are fat-based molecules that the body breaks down when it is using fat as its energy source. When used as a suffix, "genic" means "causing, forming, or producing." So, we put these terms together, and we have "ketogenic," or simply put, "causing fat burn." Ergo, the theory behind ketogenic dieting is: when a person reduces the amount of sugar and carbohydrates they consume, the body will begin to breakdown fat it already has in stores all over the body. When your body is cashing in on these stores, it is in a ketogenic state, or "ketosis." When your body consumes food, it naturally seeks carbohydrates for the purpose of breaking them down and using them as fuel. Adversely, a ketogenic cleanse trains your body to use fats for energy instead. This is achieved by lowering the amount of ingested carbohydrates and increasing the amount of ingested fats, which in turn boosts your metabolism.

Only recently has a low carb- high-fat diet plan emerged into the public eye. It is a sharp contrast to the traditional dieting style that emphasizes calorie counting. For many years it was overlooked that crash diets neglect the most important aspect of dieting: food is fuel. A diet is not meant to be treated as a once a year go to method in order to shed holiday weight in January. Rather, a diet is a lifestyle; it is a consistent pattern of how individual fuels their body. A ten day ketogenic cleanse is the perfect way to begin forming healthy eating habits that over time become second nature. If you are tired of losing weight just to gain it all back, never fear. We firmly believe that you can accomplish anything you put your mind to, including living a healthy life! You, like hundreds of others, can successfully accomplish a ketogenic cleanse and change the way you see health, fitness, and life along the way. So let's hit the books and get that metabolism working!

Benefits of Cleansing

In addition to increased metabolism and fat loss, ketogenic cleansing allows your body naturally rid itself of harmful toxins and wasteful substances. In today's modern world, food is overrun and polluted by genetically modified hormones, artificial flavors and coloring, and copious amounts of unnecessary sugars. Ketogenic cleansing eliminates bread, grains, and many other foods that are most affected by today's modern industrialization. Due to the high amount of naturally occurring foods used in a ketogenic cleanse, the body is able to obtain many vitamins and minerals that are not prevalent in a high carb diet. When the body is consuming sufficient amounts of necessary vitamins and minerals, it is able to heal itself and maintain a healthy immune system. Cleansing your body is one of the best ways to achieve, and maintain pristine health.

Chapter 2: Meal Plan Madness

One of the best ways to stay motivated, when dieting, is to find a meal plan that is easy to follow and easy on the budget. Ketogenic meals are designed to be filling while keeping within the perimeters of low-carb, high-fat guidelines. Ideally, you want to aim for 70% fats, 25% protein, and 5% carbohydrates in your diet. As long as the materials you use to build your meals are low in carbs and high in fats, feel free to experiment and find what is right for you. Each and every one of us is different, and that's okay. After all, this meal plan is for YOU!

Below is a ten-day meal plan, designed with a busy schedule in mind, which will not break the bank! All of these meals can be prepared in 30 minutes or less, and many of them are much quicker than that! There is also a list of ingredients for each meal located in the recipe chapter so you can go to the grocery store knowing exactly what you need!

	Breakfast	**Lunch**	**Dinner**
Day 1	**California Chicken Omelet** • Fat: 32 grams • 10 minutes to prepare • Protein: 25 grams • 10 minutes of cooking • Net carbs: 4 grams	**Cobb Salad** • Fat: 48 grams • 10 minutes to prepare • Protein: 43 grams • 0 minutes of cooking • Net carbs: 3 grams	**Chicken Peanut Pad Thai** • Fat: 12 grams • 15 minutes to prepare • Protein: 30 grams • 15 minutes of cooking • Net carbs: 2 g
Day 2	**Easy Blender Pancakes** • Fat: 29 grams • 5 minutes to prepare • Protein: 41 grams • 10 minutes of cooking • Net carbs: 4 grams	**Sardine Stuffed Avocados** • Fat: 29 grams • 10 minutes to prepare • Protein: 27 grams • 0 minutes of cooking	**Chipotle Fish Tacos** • Fat: 20 grams • 5 minutes to prepare • Protein: 24 grams • 15 minutes of cooking • Net carbs: 5

		• Net Carbs: 5 grams	grams
Day 3	**Steak and Eggs** • Fat: 36 grams • 10 minutes to prepare • Protein: 47 grams • 5 minutes of cooking • Net carbs: 3 grams	**Low-Carb Smoothie Bowl** • Fat 35 grams • 5 minutes to prepare • Protein: 20 grams • 0 minutes of cooking • Net carbs: 5 grams	**Avocado Lime Salmon** • Fat: 27 grams • 20 minutes to prepare • Protein: 37 grams • 10 minutes of cooking • Net carbs: 5 grams
KEEP IT UP!!!	During the course of your plan, especially around days 3 and 4, you may begin to feel like you don't have it in you. You may have thoughts telling you that you cannot last for ten days on this type pf cleanse. Do not allow feelings of discouragement bother you because, guess what? We all feel that way sometimes! A ketogenic diet causes your body to process energy like it never has before. Keep pressing on! Your body will thank you and so will you!		
Day 4	**Low-Carb Smoothie Bowl** • Fat: 35 grams • 5 minutes to prepare • Protein: 35 grams • 0 minutes of cooking • Net carbs: 4 grams	**Pesto Chicken Salad** • Fat: 27 grams • 5 minutes to prepare • Protein: 27 grams • 10 minutes of cooking • Net carbs: 3 g	**Siracha Lime Flank Steak** • Fat: 32 grams • 5 minutes to prepare • Protein: 48 grams • 10 minutes of cooking • Net Carbs: 5 g
Day 5	**Feta and Pesto Omelet** • Fat: 46 grams • 5 minutes of preparation	**Roasted Brussel Sprouts** • Fat: 21 grams • 5 minutes to prepare	**Low carb Sesame Chicken** • Fat: 36 grams • 15 minutes to prepare • Protein: 41

	• Protein: 30 grams • 5 minutes of cooking • Net carbs: 2.5 grams	• Protein: 21 grams • 30 minutes of cooking • Net carbs: 4 grams	grams • 15 minutes of cooking • Net carbs: 4 grams
Day 6	**Raspberry Cream Crepes** • Fat: 40 grams • 5 minutes of preparation • Net carbs: 8 grams • 15 minutes of cooking • Protein 15 grams	**Shakshuka** • Fat: 34 grams • Protein 35 grams • Net carbs: 4 grams • 10 minutes of preparation • 10 minutes of cooking	**Sausage in a Pan** • Fat: 38 grams • 10 minutes of preparation • Protein: 30 grams • 25 minutes of cooking • Net Carbs: 4 grams
Day 7	**Green Monster Smoothie** • Fat: 25 grams • 5 minutes of preparation • Protein: 30 grams • 0 minutes of cooking • Net Carbs: 3 grams	**Tuna Tartare** • Fat: 24 grams • 15 minutes of preparation • Protein: 56 grams • 0 minutes of cooking • Net Carbs: 4 grams	**Pesto Chicken Salad** • Fat: 27 grams • 5 minutes of preparation • Protein: 27 grams • 10 minutes of cooking • Net carbs: 3 grams
ALMOST THERE!!	By now, you can be certain you are seeing physical results such as reduced body fat and more energy! You are doing a fantastic job and you only have three days left! Keep up the good work, you owe it to yourself.		
Day 8	**Shakshuka** • Fat: 34 grams • 10 minutes of preparation	**Grilled Halloumi Salad** • Fat: 47 grams • 15 minutes of	**Keto Quarter Pounder** • Fat: 34 grams • 10 minutes of preparation

	• Protein 35 grams • 10 minutes of cooking • Net carbs: 4 grams	preparation • Protein: 21 grams • 0 minutes of cooking • Net carbs: 2 grams	• Protein: 25 grams • 8 minutes of cooking • Net carbs: 4 grams
Day 9	**Easy Blender Pancakes** • Fat: 29 grams • 5 minutes of preparation • Protein: 41 grams • 10 minutes of cooking • Net carbs: 4 grams	**Broccoli Bacon Salad** • Fat: 31 grams • 15 minutes of preparation • Protein: 10 grams • 6 minutes of cooking • Net carbs: 5 grams	**Sardine Stuffed Avocados** • Fat: 29 grams • 10 minutes to prepare • Protein: 27 grams • 0 minutes to cook • Net Carbs: 5 grams
Day 10	**California Chicken Omelet** • Fat 32 grams • 10 minutes to prepare • Protein 25 grams • 10 minutes of cooking • Net carb: 3 grams	**Shrimp Scampi** • Fat: 21 grams • 5 minutes to prepare • Protein: 21 grams • 30 minutes of cooking • Net carbs: 4 grams	**Tuna Tartare** • Fat: 36 grams • 15 minutes to prepare • Protein: 41 grams • 15 minutes of cooking • Net carbs: 4 grams
YOU DID IT!!	Congratulations! You have successfully completed a 10 day ketogenic cleanse. By now your body has adjusted to its new source of energy, expelled dozens of harmful toxins, and replenished itself with many vitamins and minerals it may have been lacking. Way to go on a job well done!		

Chapter 3: Breakfast Is For Champions

Breakfast is by far the most important meal of the day for one reason: it set the tone for the rest of your day. In order to hit the ground running, it is vital that one starts each day with foods that fuel an energetic and productive day. This chapter contains ten ketogenic breakfast ides that will have you burning fat and conquering your day like you never imagined.

1. California Chicken Omelet

- This recipe requires 10 minutes of preparation, 10 minutes of cooking time and serves 1
- Net carbs: 4 grams
- Protein: 25 grams
- Fat : 32 grams

What you will need:

- Mayo (1 tablespoon)
- Mustard (1 teaspoon)
- Campari tomato
- Eggs (2 large beaten)
- Avocado (one fourth, sliced)
- Bacon (2 slices cooked and chopped)
- Deli chicken (1 ounce)

What to do:

1. Place a skillet on the stove over a burner set to a medium heat and let it warm before adding in the eggs and seasoning as needed.
2. Once eggs are cooked about halfway through, add bacon, chicken, avocado, tomato, mayo, and mustard on one side of the eggs.
3. Fold the omelet onto its self, cover and cook for 5 additional minutes.

4. Once eggs are fully cooked and all ingredients are warm, through the center, your omelet is ready.

5. Bon apatite!

2. Steak and Eggs with Avocado

- This recipe requires 10 minutes of preparation, 5 minutes of cooking time and serves 1
- Net Carbs: 3 grams
- Protein: 44 grams
- Fat: 36 grams

What you will need:

- Salt and pepper
- Avocado (one fourth, sliced)
- Sirloin steak (4 ounce)
- Eggs (3 large)
- Butter (1 tablespoon)

What to do:

1. Melt the tablespoon of butter in a pan and fry all 3 eggs to desired doneness. Season the eggs with salt and pepper.
2. In a different pan, cook the sirloin steak to your preferred taste and slice it into thin strips. Season the steak with salt and pepper.
3. Sever your prepared steak and eggs with slices of avocado.
4. Enjoy!

3. Pancakes an a Blender

- This recipe requires 5 minutes of preparation, 10 minutes of cooking time and serves 1
- Net Carbs: 4 grams
- Protein: 41 grams
- Fat: 29 grams

What you will need:

- Whey protein powder (1 scoop)
- Eggs (2 large)
- Cream cheese (2 ounces)
- Just a pinch of cinnamon and a pinch of salt

What to do:

1. Combine cream cheese, eggs, protein powder, cinnamon, and salt into a blender. Blend for 10 seconds and let stand.
2. While letting batter stand, warm a skillet over medium heat.
3. Pour about ¼ of the batter onto warmed skillet and let cook. When bubbles begin to emerge on the surface, flip the pancake.
4. Once flipped, cook for 15 seconds. Repeat until remainder of the batter is used up.
5. Top with butter and/ or sugar- free maple syrup and you are all set!
6. Chow time!

4. Low Carb Smoothe Bowl

- Net Carbs: 4 grams

- Protein: 35 grams

- Fat: 35 grams

- Takes 5 minutes to prepare and serves 1.

What you will need:

- Spinach (1 cup)

- Almond milk (half a cup)

- Coconut oil (1 tablespoon)

- Low carb protein powder (1 scoop)

- Ice cubes (2 cubes)

- Whipping cream (2 T)

- Optional toppings can include: raspberries, walnuts, shredded coconut, or chia seeds

What to do:

1. Place spinach in blender. Add almond milk, cream, coconut oil, and ice. Blend until thoroughly and evenly combined.

2. Pour into bowl.

3. Top with toppings or stir lightly into smoothie.

4. Treat yourself!

5. Feta and Pesto Omelet

- This recipe requires 5 minutes of preparation, 5 minutes of cooking time and serves 1
- Net Carbs: 2.5 grams
- Protein: 30 grams
- Fat: 46 grams

What you will need:

- Butter (1 tablespoon)
- Eggs (3 large)
- Heavy cream (1 tablespoon)
- Feta cheese (1 ounce)
- Basil pesto (1 teaspoon)
- Tomatoes (optional)

What to do:

1. Heat pan and melt butter.
2. Beat eggs together with heavy whipping cream (will give eggs a fluffy consistency once cooked).
3. Pour eggs in pan and cook until almost done, add feta and pesto to on half of eggs.
4. Fold omelet and cook for an additional 4-5 minutes.
5. Top with feta and tomatoes, and eat up!

6. Crepes with Cream and Raspberries

- This recipe requires 5 minutes of preparation, 15 minutes of cooking time and serves 2
- Net Carbs: 8 grams
- Protein: 15 grams
- Fat: 40 grams

What you will need:

- Raspberries (3 ounces, fresh or frozen)
- Whole Milk Ricotta (half a cup and 2 tablespoons)
- Erythritol (2 tablespoons)
- Eggs (2 large)
- Cream Cheese (2 ounces)
- Pinch of salt
- Dash of Cinnamon
- Whipped cream and sugar- free maple syrup to go on top

What to do:

1. In a blender, blend cream cheese, eggs, erythritol, salt, and cinnamon for about 20 seconds, or until there are no lumps of cream cheese.
2. Place a pan on a burner turned to a medium heat before coating in cooking spray. Add 20 percent of your batter to the pan in a thin layer. Cook crepe until the underside becomes slightly darkened. Carefully flip the crepe and let the reverse side cook for about 15 seconds.
3. Repeat step 3 until all batter is used.
4. Without stacking the crepes, allow them to cool for a few minutes.
5. After the crepes have cool, place about 2 tablespoons of ricotta cheese in the center of each crepe.
6. Throw in a couple of raspberries and fold the side to the middle.
7. Top those off with some whipped cream and sugar- free maple syrup and…

8. Viola! You're a true chef! Indulge in your creation!

7. Green Monster Smoothie

- This recipe requires 10 minutes of preparation, 0 minutes of cooking time and serves 1
- Net Carbs: 4 grams
- Protein: 30 grams
- Fat: 25 grams

What you will need:

- Almond milk (one and a half cups)
- Spinach (one eighth of a cup)
- Cucumber (fourth of a cup)
- Celery (fourth of a cup)
- Avocado (fourth of a cup)
- Coconut oil (1 tablespoon)
- Stevia (liquid, 10 drops)
- Whey Protein Powder (1 scoop)

What to do:

1. In a blender, blend almond milk and spinach for a few pulses.
2. Add remaining ingredients and blend until thoroughly combined.

- Add optional matcha powder, if desired, and enjoy!

Chapter 4: Lunch Crunch

Eating a healthy lunch when you are limited on time due to, work, school, or taking care of your kids can be a tumultuous task. Thankfully, we have compiled a list of eight quick and easy recipes to accompany the ten day meal plan laid out in chapter 2! Many find it advantageous, especially if you work throughout the week, to prepare you meals ahead of time. Thankfully, these lunch recipes are also easy to pack and take on the go!

1. Off The Cobb Salad

- Net carbs: 3 grams
- Protein: 43 grams
- Fat: 48 grams
- Takes 10 minutes to prepare and serves 1.

What you will need:
- Spinach (1 cup)
- Egg (1, hard-boiled)
- Bacon (2 strips)
- Chicken breast (2 ounces)
- Campari tomato (one half of tomato)
- Avocado (one fourth, sliced)
- White vinegar (half of a teaspoon)
- Olive oil (1 tablespoon)

What to do:
1. Cook chicken and bacon completely and cut or slice into small pieces.
2. Chop remaining ingredients into bite size pieces.
3. Place all ingredients, including chicken and bacon, in a bowl, toss ingredients in oil and vinegar.
4. Enjoy!

2. Avocado and Sardines

- Net Carbs: 5 grams
- Protein: 27 grams
- Fat: 52 grams
- Takes 10 minutes to prepare and serves 1.

What you will need:

- Fresh lemon juice (1 tablespoon)
- Spring onion or chives (1 or small bunch)
- Mayonnaise (1 tablespoon)
- Sardines (1 tin, drained)
- Avocado (1 whole, seed removed)
- Turmeric powder (fourth of a teaspoon) or freshly ground turmeric root (1 teaspoon)
- Salt (fourth of a teaspoon)

What to do:

1. Begin by cutting the avocado in half and removing its seed.
2. Scoop out about half the avocado and set aside (shown below).
3. In small bowl, mash drained sardines with fork.
4. Add onion (or chives), turmeric powder, and mayonnaise. Mix well.
5. Add removed avocado to sardine mixture.
6. Add lemon juice and salt.
7. Scoop the mixture into avocado halves.
8. Dig   in!

3. Chicken Salad A La Pesto

- This recipe requires 5minutes of preparation, 10 minutes of cooking time and serves 4
- Net Carbs: 3 grams
- Protein: 27 grams
- Fat: 27 grams

What you will need:

- Garlic pesto (2 tablespoons)
- Mayonnaise (fourth of a cup)
- Grape tomatoes (10, halved)
- Avocado (1, cubed)
- Bacon (6 slices, cooked crisp and crumbled)
- Chicken (1 pound, cooked and cubed)
- Romaine lettuce (optional)

What to do:

1. Combine all ingredients in a large mixing bowl.
2. Toss gently to spread mayonnaise and pesto evenly throughout.
3. If desired, wrap in romaine lettuce for a low-carb BLT chicken wrap.
4. Bon apatite!

4. Bacon and Roasted Brussel Sprouts

- This recipe requires 5 minutes of preparation, 30 minutes of cooking time and serves 4
- Net Carbs: 4 grams
- Protein: 15 grams
- Fat: 21 grams

What you will need:

- Bacon (8 strips)

117

- Olive oil (2 tablespoons)
- Brussel sprouts (1 pound, halved)
- Salt and pepper

What to do:

1. Preheat oven to 375 degrees Fahrenheit.

2. Gently mix Brussel sprouts with olive oil, salt, and pepper.

3. Spread Brussel sprouts evenly onto a greased baking sheet.

4. Bake in oven for 30 minutes. Shake the pan about halfway through to mix the Brussel sprout halves up a bit.

5. While Brussel sprouts are in the oven, fry bacon slices on stovetop.

6. When bacon is fully cooked, let cool and chop it into bite size pieces.

7. Combine bacon and Brussel sprouts in a bowl and you're finished!

8. Feast!!

5. Grilled Halloumi Salad

- Net Carbs: 7 grams
- Protein: 21 grams
- Fat: 47 grams
- Takes 15 minutes to prepare and serves 1.

What you will need:

- Chopped walnuts (half of an ounce)
- Baby arugula (1 handful)
- Grape tomatoes (5)
- Cucumber (1)
- Halloumi cheese (3 ounces)
- Olive oil (1 teaspoon)
- Balsamic vinegar (half of a teaspoon)
- A pinch of salt

What to do:

1. Slice halloumi cheese into slices 1/3 of an in thick.
2. Grill cheese for 3 to 5 minutes, until you see grill lines, on each side.
3. Wash and cut veggies into bite size pieces, place in salad bowl.
4. Add rinsed baby arugula and walnuts to veggies.
5. Toss in olive oil, balsamic vinegar, and salt.
6. Place grilled halloumi on top of veggies and your lunch is ready!
7. Eat those greens and get back to work!

6. Bacon Broccoli Salad

- This recipe requires 15 minutes of preparation, 6 minutes of cooking time and serves 5.
- Net Carbs: 5 grams
- Protein: 10 grams
- Fat: 31 grams

What you will need:

- Sesame oil (half of a teaspoon)
- Erythritol (1 and a half tablespoons) or stevia to taste
- White vinegar (1 tablespoon)
- Mayonnaise (half of a cup)
- Green onion (three fourths of an ounce)
- Bacon (fourth of a pound)
- Broccoli (1 pound, heads and stalks cut and trimmed)

What to do:

1. Cook bacon and crumble into bits.
2. Cut broccoli into bite sized pieces.
3. Slice scallions.
4. Mix mayonnaise, vinegar, erythritol (or stevia), and sesame oil, to make the dressing.
5. Place broccoli and bacon bits in a bowl and toss with dressing.
6. Viola!

7. Tuna Avocado Tartare

- Net Carbs: 4 grams
- Protein: 56 grams
- Fat: 24 grams
- Takes 15 minutes to prepare and serves 2.

What you will need:

- Sesame seed oil (2 tablespoons)
- Sesame seeds (1 teaspoon)
- Cucumbers (2)
- Lime (half of a whole lime)
- Mayonnaise (1 tablespoon)
- Sriracha (1 tablespoon)
- Olive oil (2 tablespoons)
- Jalapeno (one half of whole jalapeno)
- Scallion (3 stalks)
- Avocado (1)
- Tuna steak (1 pound)
- Soy sauce (1 tablespoon)

What to do:

1. Dice tuna and avocado into ¼ inch cubes, place in bowl.

2. Finely chop scallion and jalapeno, add to bowl.

3. Pour olive oil, sesame oil, siracha, soy sauce, mayonnaise, and lime into bowl.

4. Using hands, toss all ingredients to combine evenly. Using a utensil may breakdown avocado, which you want to remain chunky, so it is best to use your hands.

5. Top with sesame seeds and serve with a side of sliced cucumber.

6. There's certainly something fishy about this recipe, but it tastes great! Enjoy!

8. Warm Spinach and Shrimp

- This recipe requires 15 minutes of preparation, 6 minutes of cooking time and serves 5.

- Fat: 24 grams

- Protein: 36 grams

- Net Carbs: 3 grams

- Takes10 minutes to prepare, 5 minutes to cook, and serves 2.

What you will need:

- Spinach (2 handfuls)

- Parmesan (half a tablespoon)

- Heavy cream (1 tablespoon)

- Olive oil (1 tablespoon)

- Butter (2 tablespoons)

- Garlic (3 cloves)

- Onion (one fourth of whole onion)

- Large raw shrimp (about 20)

- Lemon (optional)

What to do:

1. Place peeled shrimp in cold water.

2. Chop onions and garlic into fine pieces.

3. Heat oil, in pan, over medium heat. Cook shrimp in oil until lightly pink (we do not want them fully cooked here). Remove shrimp from oil and set aside.

4. Place chopped onions and garlic into pan, cook until onions are translucent. Add a dash of salt.

5. Add butter, cream, and parmesan cheese. Stir until you have a smooth sauce.

6. Let sauce cook for about 2 minutes so it will thicken slightly.

7. Place shrimp back into pan and cook until done. This should take no longer than 2 or 3 minutes. Be careful not to overcook the shrimp, it will become dry and tough!

8. Remove shrimp and sauce from pan and replace with spinach. Cook spinach VERY briefly

9. Place warmed spinach onto a plate.

10. Pour shrimp and sauce over bed of spinach, squeeze some lemon on top, if you like, and you're ready to chow down!

Chapter 5: Thinner by Dinner

It's the end of the day and you are winding down from a hard day's work. Your body does not require a lot of energy while you sleep; therefore, dinner will typically consist of less fat and more protein.

1. Chicken Pad Thai

- Net Carbs: 7 grams
- Protein: 30 grams
- Fat: 12 grams
- Takes 15 minutes to prepare, 15 minutes to cook, and serves 4.

What you will need:

- Peanuts (1 ounce)
- Lime (1 whole)
- Soy sauce (2 tablespoons)
- Egg (1 large)
- Zucchini (2 large)
- Chicken thighs (16 ounces, boneless and skinless)
- Garlic (2 cloves, minced)
- White onion (1,chopped)
- Olive oil (1 tablespoon)
- Chili flakes (optional)

What to do:

1. Over medium heat, cook olive oil and onion until translucent. Add the garlic and cook about three minutes (until fragrant).
2. Cook chicken in pan for 5 to 7 minutes on each side (until fully cooked). Remove chicken from heat and shred it using a couple of forks.
3. Cut ends off zucchini and cut into thin noodles. Set zucchini noodles aside.
4. Next, scramble the egg in the pan.

5. Once the egg is fully cooked, and the zucchini noodles and cook for about 2 minutes.

6. Add the previously shredded chicken to the pan.

7. Give it some zing with soy sauce, lime juice, peanuts, and chili flakes.

8. Time to eat!

2. Chipotle Style Fish Tacos

- Fat: 20 grams

- Protein: 24 grams

- Net Carbs: 7 grams

- Takes 5 minutes to prepare, 15 minutes to cook, and serves 4.

What you will need:

- Low carb tortillas (4)
- Haddock fillets (1 pound)
- Mayonnaise (2 tablespoons)
- Butter (2 tablespoons)
- Chipotle peppers in adobo sauce (4 ounces)
- Garlic (2 cloves, pressed)
- Jalapeño (1 fresh, chopped)
- Olive oil (2 tablespoons)
- Yellow onion (half of an onion, diced)

What to do:

1. Fry diced onion (until translucent) in olive oil in a high sided pan, over medium- high heat.

2. Reduce heat to medium, add jalapeno and garlic. Cook while stir for another two minutes.

3. Chop the chipotle peppers and add them, along with the adobo sauce, to the pan.

4. Add the butter, mayo, and fish fillets to the pan.

5. Cook the fish fully while breaking up the fillets and stirring the fish into other ingredients.

6. Warm tortillas for 2 minutes on each side.

7. Fill tortillas with fishy goodness and eat up!

3. Salmon with Avocado Lime Sauce

- Net Carbs: 5 grams
- Protein: 37 grams
- Fat: 27 grams
- Takes 20 minutes to prepare, 10 minutes to cook, and serves 2.

What you will need:

- Salmon (two 6 ounce fillets)
- Avocado (1 large)
- Lime (one half of a whole lime)
- Red onion (2 tablespoons, diced)
- Cauliflower (100 grams)

What to do:

1. Chop cauliflower in a blender or food processor then cook it in a lightly oiled pan, while covered, for 8 minutes. This will make the cauliflower rice-like.
2. Next, blend the avocado with squeezed lime juice in the blender or processor until smooth and creamy.
3. Heat some oil in a skillet and cook salmon (skin side down first) for 4 to 5 minute. Flip the fillets and cook for an additional 4 to 5 minutes.
4. Place salmon fillet on a bed of your cauliflower rice and top with some diced red onion.

4. Siracha Lime Steak

- Net Carbs: 5 grams
- Protein: 48 grams
- Fat: 32 grams
- Takes 5 minutes to prepare, 10 minutes to cook, and serves 2.

What you will need:

- Vinegar (1 teaspoon)
- Olive oil (2 tablespoons)
- Lime (1 whole)
- Sriracha (2 tablespoons)
- Flank steak (16 ounce)
- Salt and pepper

What to do:

1. Season steak, liberally, with salt and pepper. Place on baking sheet, lined with foil, and broil in oven for 5 minutes on each side (add another minute or two for a well done steak). Remove from oven, cover, and set aside.
2. Place sriracha in small bowl and squeeze lime into it. Whisk in salt, pepper, and vinegar.
3. Slowly pour in olive oil.
4. Slice steak into thin slices, lather on your sauce, and enjoy!
5. Feel free to pair this recipe with a side of greens such as asparagus or broccoli.

5. Low Carb Sesame Chicken

- Net Carbs: 4 grams

- Protein: 45 grams

- Fat: 36 grams

- Takes 15minutes to prepare, 15 minutes to cook, and serves 2.

What you will need:

- Broccoli (three fourths of a cup, cut bite size)

- Xanthan gum (fourth of a teaspoon)

- Sesame seeds (2 tablespoons)

- Garlic (1 clove)

- Ginger (1 cm cube)

- Vinegar (1 tablespoon)

- Brown sugar alternative (Sukrin Gold is a good one) (2 tablespoons)

- Soy sauce (2 tablespoons)

- Toasted sesame seed oil (2 tablespoons)

- Arrowroot powder or corn starch (1 tablespoon)

- Chicken thighs (1poundcut into bite sized pieces)

- Egg (1 large)

- Salt and pepper

- Chives (optional)

What to do:

1. First we will make the batter by combining the egg with a tablespoon of arrowroot powder (or cornstarch). Whisk well.

2. Place chicken pieces in batter. Be sure to coat all sides of chicken pieces with the batter.

3. Heat one tablespoon of sesame oil, in a large pan. Add chicken pieces to hot oil and fry. Be gentle when flipping the chicken, you want to keep the batter from falling off. It should take about 10 minutes for them to cook fully.

4. Next, make the sesame sauce. In a small bowl, combine soy sauce, brown sugar alternative, vinegar, ginger, garlic, sesame seeds, and the remaining tablespoon of toasted sesame seed oil. Whisk very well.

5. Once the chicken is fully cooked, add broccoli and the sesame sauce to pan and cook for an additional 5 minutes.

6. Spoon desired amount into a bowl, top it off with some chopped chives, and relish in some fine dining at home!

6. Pan 'O Sausage

- Net Carbs: 4 grams

- Protein: 30 grams

- Fat: 38 grams

- Takes 10 minutes to prepare, 25 minutes to cook, and serves 2.

What you will need:

- Basil (half a teaspoon)

- Oregano (half a teaspoon)

- White onion (1 tablespoon)

- Shredded mozzarella (fourth of a cup)

- Parmesan cheese (fourth of a cup)

- Vodka sauce (half a cup)

- Mushrooms (4 ounces)

- Sausage (3 links)

- Salt (fourth of a teaspoon)

- Red pepper (fourth of a teaspoon, ground)

What to do:

1. Preheat oven to 350 degrees Fahrenheit.

2. Heat an iron skillet over medium flame. When skillet is hot, cook sausage links until almost thoroughly cooked.

3. While sausage is cooking, slice mushrooms and onion.

4. When sausage is almost fully cooked, remove links from heat and place mushrooms and onions in skillet to brown.

5. Cut sausage into pieces about ½ inch thick and place pieces in pan.

6. Season skillet contents with oregano, basil, salt, and red pepper.

7. Add vodka sauce and parmesan cheese. Stir everything together.

8. Place skillet in oven for 15 minutes. Sprinkle mozzarella on top a couple minutes before removing dish from oven.

9. Once 15 minutes is up, remove skillet from the oven and let cool for a few minutes.

10. Dinner   time!

7. Quarter Pounder Keto Burger

- Net Carbs: 4 grams

- Protein: 25 grams

- Fat: 34 grams

- Takes 10 minutes to prepare, 8 minutes to cook, and serves 2.

What you will need:

- Basil (half a teaspoon)
- Cayenne (fourth a teaspoon)
- Crushed red pepper (half a teaspoon)
- Salt (half a teaspoon)
- Lettuce (2 large leaves)
- Butter (2 tablespoons)
- Egg (1 large)
- Sriracha (1 tablespoon)
- Onion (fourth of whole onion)
- Plum tomato (half of whole tomato)
- Mayo (1 tablespoon)
- Pickled jalapenos (1 tablespoon, sliced)
- Bacon (1 strip)
- Ground beef (half a pound)
- Bacon (1 strip)

What to do:

1. Knead mean for about three minute.
2. Chop bacon, jalapeno, tomato, and onion into fine pieces. (shown below)
3. Knead in mayo, sriracha, egg, and chopped ingredients, and spices into meat.
4. Separate meat into four even pieces and flatten them (not thinly, just press on the tops to create a flat surface). Place a tablespoon of butter on top of two of the meat pieces. Take the pieces that do not have butter of them and set them

on top of the buttered ones (basically creating a butter and meat sandwich). Seal the sides together, concealing the butter within.

5. Throw the patties on the grill (or in a pan) for about 5 minutes on each side. Caramelize some onions if you want too!

6. Prepare large leaves of lettuce by spreading some mayo onto them. Once patties are finished, place them on one half of the lettuce, add your desired burger toppings, and fold the other half over of the lettuce leaf over the patty.

Burger time!

BREAKFAST

Breakfast Recipes To Start Your Day Strong

Sconey Sconey Sunday – 6 SmartPoints Per Serving

This breakfast dish is best made on the weekend and enjoyed all week long. This breakfast should be filling in the moment due to the fluffiness of the scone and should keep you satisfied all morning because of the liberal use of peaches. If you are new to baking, or just a little bit afraid of your own oven, this is a great recipe to start with. There is no need to wait for any ingredients to rise and it builds the foundation for many other scone recipes. You can replace the peach with blueberries, banana, apple, etc. Try and experiment to find what you like most.

Ready in 25 Minutes

10 minutes to prep and 15 minutes to cook

Ingredients (serves 4):

2/3 cups of all purpose flour

½ teaspoon of baking powder

½ teaspoon of baking soda

1 teaspoon of powdered sugar

2 tablespoons of sugar

½ teaspoon of half and half

1 teaspoon of margarine

1/3 cup of vanilla yogurt (I highly recommend Stoneyfield for the best results)

1 teaspoon of salt

3 tablespoons of chopped peaches (if you are using canned peaches, make sure you drain the peaches and give the peaches some time to dry. I recommend not using canned as they tend to contain additional sugars that add unnecessary calories and distort the flavor of the peaches)

Non-stick cooking spray

Step 1:

Preheat the oven to 400 degrees F or 205 degrees C

Step 2:

Take a medium size mixing bowl and add the flour, sugar (not powdered), baking powder, baking soda, and salt. Mix the ingredients and add in the margarine while doing so. The margarine can be difficult to work with so you may want to heat it up in a microwave for 15 seconds, or alternatively cut the margarine into small pieces. Only move onto step 4 when you have a consistent base in the bowl – the margarine should be fully mixed in.

Step 3:

Add the yogurt and the peaches, mixing while you do so.

Step 4:

Take a large piece of wax paper and empty the contents of the bowl onto the paper. Knead the dough for 3-4 minutes. Many are unsure of how to knead the dough, so think about it as folding the dough over itself over and over.

Step 5:

Coat a large baking tray with non-stick spray and form the scones on the tray. The scones look best when shaped like triangles. The exact size of the scones is not as important as making sure the scones are of equal size. This recipe usually yields between 4 and 6 scones. Make sure the dough is firmly pressed against the baking tray. Bake for 12-15 minutes on the center oven rack.

Step 6:

Remove the scones from the oven and while still hot, paint the scones with milk. This should look like they are slightly moist from the milk. Use this moisture to spread the powdered sugar over the scones. You can serve these right away and they will last about one week at room temperature.

10 Minute Fried Toast – 3 SmartPoints Per Serving

Yes this recipe is truly just a variation of French Toast but I want to stress the importance of a hot breakfast and that it doesn't take too much time to prepare one. This dish can be enjoyed even on a weekday before work and with a little practice you can cut down on the prep time dramatically. This is a dish I commonly make for my daughter before school and it can be made almost as fast as some simple scrambled eggs.

Ready in 10 Minutes

5 minutes to prep and 5 minutes to cook

Ingredients (serves 2):

4 egg whites

6 slices of wheat bread (you'll have lots of options of bread but I suggest looking at the low calorie version. I have switched to 40-45 calorie bread per slice and haven't noticed a big difference. The slices are a little smaller but each piece is less than half the calories of traditional white bread)

¼ cup of 1% milk

2 tablespoons of sugar free maple syrup (this recipe changes to 5 SmartPoints per serving with regular syrup)

1 tablespoon of cinnamon

1 tablespoon of vanilla extract

Non-stick cooking spray

Step 1:

In a shallow mixing bowl, add the egg whites, milk, and vanilla extract. Whisk these ingredients together.

Step 2:

Coat a skillet with cooking spray and put it over low-medium heat. Dip both sides of your wheat bread into the mixing bowl from step 1 and add to the skillet. You should be able to cook roughly 2 pieces at a time.

Step 3:

While still hot, sprinkle cinnamon on each piece of toast. Serve with syrup and enjoy right away.

3 Minute Breakfast Mug – 2 SmartPoints Per Serving

Perhaps you thought 10 minutes was too long to dedicate to cooking a warm breakfast, well then this recipe is for you. This is a breakfast I used to make at the office as the ingredients can be stored easily in a refrigerator. You will absolutely need to use the liquid egg substitute as opposed to liquid eggs as the substitute will cook better in the microwave. If you have never used your microwave as a primary cooking tool, do not fear – this too was my first recipe cooked entirely in a microwave. When you get a look at the finished product you will be highly satisfied with the result – it tastes great too.

Ready in 3 Minutes

1 minute to prep and 2 minutes to cook

Ingredients (serves 1):

½ cup of liquid egg substitute

1 ounce of low-fat turkey breast (optional)

1 slice of American cheese

Non-stick cooking spray

Step 1:

Take a microwave-safe mug and coat it with the non-stick spray.

Step 2:

Pour the egg substitute into the mug and microwave on high for 1 minute.

Step 3:

Add in the cheese and optionally the turkey. If you're adding the turkey, you will want to make sure that it is in very fine pieces. Microwave for an additional minute.

Saturday Morning Enriching Oatmeal – 7 SmartPoints

This filling breakfast will have you thinking differently about oatmeal. We take a hearty essential oatmeal recipe and add a combination of zesty flavors that make the dish shine. This breakfast takes longer than the others to cook and is best enjoyed on a weekend, or when you have some extra time before starting your day. This recipe can easily be doubled or tripled to serve the entire family.

Ready in 30 Minutes

10 minutes to prep and 20 minutes to cook

Ingredients (serves 1):

½ cup raw oats

2 teaspoons of lemon juice

1/8 teaspoon of cinnamon

1/8 teaspoon of salt

1 low-calorie sweetener packet similar to Splenda

1 cup of unsweetened almond milk, or vanilla soy milk

1 cup of water

Step 1:

In a small pot, combine the oats, cinnamon, salt, almond milk, and water.

Step 2:

Heat the pot on high heat and bring the oatmeal to a near boil. Once bubbling reduce the heat to low. Cook for 10-15 minutes after the oatmeal has been put to low heat.

Step 3:

Stir occasionally and remove from burner when the oatmeal has thickened.

Step 4:

Before serving, add the sweetener packet to the serving bowl.

LUNCH RECIPES THAT WILL KEEP YOU SATISFIED ALL AFTERNOON

Home Joe's Mediterranean Hummus With Pita Bread – 4 Smart Points Per Serving

This recipe is based on a small love affair I have for the Trader Joe's Mediterranean Hummus. I have tweaked this recipe to get very much the same taste, but with all the added benefit of knowing exactly what ingredients are used. This hummus is packed full of healthy fats from the chick peas, fats that will leave you satisfied all afternoon. I love to bring a small container to work and pair it with either pita chips or pita bread and a side of fresh vegetables – carrots and peppers in particular. Be on the lookout for the nutritional information on the chips or pita bread of your choice – while the hummus is healthy, aim for a serving of less than 200 calories for whatever you choose to dip in the hummus and add 2 smart points to the meal. Feel free to use as many veggies as you want for dipping though, think about these as 0 points.

Ready in 30 Minutes

30 minutes to prepare.

Ingredients (serves 8):

A food processor that can hold 3 cups

1 large garlic glove

2 tablespoons of tahini

½ lemon

6 tablespoons of extra virgin olive oil (the taste is important here, so use extra virgin instead of "pure")

¼ teaspoon of cumin

1 teaspoon of crushed red pepper

½ cup of boiling water

Step 0:

This recipe is dependent on your food processor. You won't need to prepare any ingredients, but make sure that your processor is up to the task. I have had this recipe come out just a tad too lumpy in the past because of the food processor, so blending time may vary slightly to get the consistency that you want.

Step 1:

Put the garlic clove and the processor and pulse 3 to 4 times. Add the rest of the ingredients except for the water.

Step 2:

Run the processor for 3-5 minutes, periodically switching from pulse to long sustained processing.

Step 3:

Pour in the hot water (does not need to be exactly boiling) and run the processor for an additional 30 seconds to a minute. Check the consistency of the hummus and run the processor for additional time if needed. You may need to add more than ½ a cup of water depending in the consistency of the beans and how powerful your food processor is.

Step 4:

With the desired consistency, pour the hummus in to a container and store in the fridge for several hours. Serving right away will not yield the best flavor as the ingredients are still settling.

Step 5 (Optional):

If serving for a party or if you simply want slightly more indulgent hummus, add a drizzle of olive oil to the hummus before serving.

5 Minute Turkey Wrap – 8 SmartPoints Per Serving

I ate these wraps nearly three times a week for half a year – they were just that delicious. They're easy to make and great to bring as a bagged lunch.

Ready in 5 Minutes

5 minutes to prep and 0 minutes to cook

Ingredients (serves 1)

3 ounces of low-sodium turkey breast (I encourage you to use your local deli counter versus the prepackaged meats – the deli counter meats will often have less sodium so even if you aren't purchasing 'low-sodium' turkey, it is probably still worth it to buy from the deli counter)

1 ounce of lettuce or spinach

¼ of one whole tomato

1 tablespoon of low-fat ranch dressing

1 ounce of low-fat mozzarella cheese (you can use other cheeses, but for the calorie to size ratio, I find mozzarella to be the best investment)

1 wrap or flatbread that is between 100-150 calories per wrap/flatbread (your supermarket will have several options for you but I suggest the Flatout Wraps. These wraps are fluffy and delicious are only 90 calories. For wraps above 150 calories, add another SmartPoint to the recipe)

Step 1:

Take out your wrap or flatbread and heat it in the microwave for 15-20 seconds – this will fluff up your wrap and make it more malleable to shape.

Step 2:

Spread your low-fat ranch dressing over the wrap. Fill the wrap with your turkey, lettuce or spinach, tomatoes, and cheese.

Step 3:

Roll up your wrap and store for lunch or eat right away.

Slow Cooker Southern Style Chicken Soup -4 SmartPoints Per Serving

It's an all day affair that that will last you all week and then some. This hearty soup is great in the winter and full of exotic blends of flavors that will have you wondering why you don't eat soup more often. Since this recipe produces a fairly large batch, it's worth noting that this soup freezes extremely well. If you decide to freeze individual servings, simply let the soup thaw at room temperature before you reheat in the microwave – this is the best way to preserve the flavor.

Ready in 7 Hours

10 minutes to prep and 6-8 hours to cook

Ingredients (serves 10)

2 large chicken breasts cut into inch size cubes

1 clove of finely minced garlic

1 cup of corn (canned is what I use)

½ diced large white onion

½ cup of finely chopped chilantro

1 teaspoon of cumin

1 tablespoon of chili powder

15 ounces of washed and drained kidney beans (canned is what I use)

15 ounces of washed and drained black beans (canned is what I use)

1 teaspoon of lime juice

2 whole bell peppers cut into long strips

1 15 ounce can of diced tomatoes

Pepper to taste

Salt to taste

Step 1:

Prepare all of your ingredients and pour them into your slow cooker. Put the slow cookers on low heat and let cook for 6-8 hours. To make sure that the soup is done, reach for a piece of chicken and slice to find the color in the center. Note that it is very difficult to overcook this recipe – even 9 hours in the slow cooker will result in a fantastic soup.

Alternative: If you do not have a slow cooker, do not fret – a regular pot on low heat on your burner will do just fine. There are some limitations however in that you will need to be present the entire time the soup is cooking. It is also possible to overcook the soup if you are using a traditional pot (I first made this recipe using this method and it turned out great. It does require time and patience if you're using a pot, but it can be made over the weekend and enjoyed all week long).

Healthy Zone Calzone – 4 SmartPoints Per Serving

I love this recipe because it uses a neat trick – we substitute heavy dough for Pillsbury and get to cut down on the cooking time in the process. This dish is great by itself and works great as a lunch served at room temperature. If you decide to make the marinara sauce in the next chapter, try it as a dipping sauce for this delicious healthy calzone.

Ready in 40 Minutes

25 minutes to prep and 15 minutes to cook

Ingredients (serves 8):

1 can of reduced fat crescent rolls by Pillsbury (this is absolutely necessary to get the right amount of dough to calorie ratio)

¼ cup of reduce fat shredded cheese (mozzarella is my go to choice but feel free to use your favorite).

6 ounces of low-fat chicken breast

2 cups of baby spinach

6 tablespoons of low-fat whipped cream cheese (you can also use reduced fat but know that it changes the total SmartPoints per serving quite significantly).

1-2 tablespoons of vegetable oil

Step 1:

Take the chicken breast and cut it into cubes before cooking in a frying pan. Use the vegetable oil to cook the chicken and try to use the least amount of oil possible. This recipe is extremely lean and the vegetable oil is actually one of the more calorie expensive ingredients – any savings here do add up.

Step 2:

Preheat the oven to 375 degrees F or 190 degrees C.

Step 3:

Remove the Pillsbury rolls and arrange them on an ungreased baking tray. The container should contain 8 rolls but we are only making 4 calzones. Combine rolls to make the 4 calzones and make sure each roll is flat on the tray.

Step 4:

Spread over each roll the baby spinach, cream cheese, chicken, and your choice of shredded cheese. These rolls are fairly small for how stuffed these calzones will be (definitely a good thing), so you may need to kneed some of the ingredients into the dough itself – this works particularly well with the cream cheese and shredded cheese.

Step 5:

Form each of the individual 4 calzones, fold the dough over the ingredients and 'close' the calzone. This step can be a little tricky if the dough is not at room temperature. The final shape should look a little bit like a crescent moon

Step 6:

Bake for 10-15 minutes in the middle rack of the oven. You will know when the calzones are ready as the dough will begin to flake and turn brown.

8 Minute Tuna – 3 SmartPoints Per Serving

I still prepare this Tuna Salad at least twice a month. It's quick and easy and great to bring to work. If you feel like you're missing out on the pure indulgence of 'fatty' flavors then this salad will hit the spot. Even though we are using low-fat mayonnaise, it still hits all the right notes and you'd be hard pressed to tell the difference between this and a much more calorie dense mayonnaise base. One of the greatest aspects of this recipe, and why it's only 3 SmartPoints per serving, is the use of lettuce as the base for wraps.

We use lettuce for a couple of reasons: one, the neutral flavor of the lettuce brings out the creaminess of the salad without distorting the taste and two, the crispness of the lettuce is essential for the proper texture. I came up with the idea for using lettuce as a base after eating Korean barbeque. Try it and you'll see how it really does bring out the flavor.

Ready in 8 Minutes

8 minutes to prep and 0 minutes to cook

Ingredients (serves 4):

12 ounces of albacore white tuna in water (essential as this tuna has the meatiest texture and taste)

3 tablespoons of low-fat mayonnaise

3 stalks o chopped celery (if any part of the stalk is not hard, then do not use that section. You want the celery to be firm as to add a crunchiness to the salad).

1 teaspoon of Dijon mustard

½ teaspoon of black pepper

½ teaspoon of table-salt (do not use sea-salt as the harsher grain does not spread as evenly throughout the salad)

½ head of lettuce cut into large pieces (these will serve as the wraps for eating the tuna so keep that in mind as you cut the lettuce)

Step 1:

Drain the tuna and add to a large mixing bowl. Add the celery, pepper, salt, mustard, and mayonnaise. Stir well, breaking up the large pieces of tuna that might be sticking together from the can.

Step 2:

For best results, leave the salad in the fridge for 20 minutes to let thicken. Serve with the large pieces of lettuce.

Week-Long Rice With Chicken – 4 SmartPoints Per Serving

One of the essentials of preparing a good lunch is not having to worry about side dishes. This dish comes with everything you need – protein to keep you full, carbohydrates to give you afternoon energy, and veggies for your general nutrition and to flavor the dish. This rice dish can be stored away for work and can be enjoyed at room temperature or even cold – it will still taste delicious!

Ready in 30 Minutes

15 minutes to prep and 15 minutes to cook

Ingredients (serves 6):

2 large lean, boneless chicken breasts

2 large eggs

2 cups uncooked brown rice

½ cup of pea

½ cup of chopped carrots

2 finely chopped cloves of garlic

2 tablespoons of soy sauce (1 tablespoon if using low-sodium soy sauce – better results are gotten with regular soy)

4 tablespoons of water

Non-stick cooking spray or if unavailable, 1 tablespoon of vegetable oil

Step 1:

Take the chicken breast and cut the chicken into long strips. The important part of cutting the chicken is that each strip has roughly the same thickness. Do not worry about how thick or thin your chicken is – just make sure it is fairy uniform.

Step 2:

Cook the brown rice on your stovetop. Use 5 cups of water for the 2 cups of brown rice. This is more water than is typically used and you will need to cook the rice for slightly longer. The rice will fluff up much more with that extra cup of water. Move onto step 3 only after the rice is done.

Step 3:

In a large skillet, scramble the two large eggs and set aside.

Step 4:

Coat the same skillet again with non-stick cooking spray. Each skillet is a little bit difference and if you know that non-stick spray is not going to be able to grease the entire pan, use 1 tablespoon of vegetable oil, as we do not want the chicken to stick to the pan. Add the sliced chicken and cook halfway before adding the carrots. As the chicken starts to look fully cooked, add the chopped garlic and peas.

Step 4:

Take the soy sauce and pour it into a small dish with the water. Mix and pour into the skillet. The water will evaporate and ensure that the soy sauce is not too overpowering. Move onto step 5 once the chicken is fully cooked and the water is mostly evaporated.

Step 5:

Add into the skillet the cooked rice and scrambled eggs. Mix well and remove from the burner once the eggs have warmed up. Serve right away.

Admiral David's Broccoli – 5 SmartPoints Per Serving

If the name seems familiar, or just a bit off, that's because it is indeed a variation of General Tso's Chicken. It's a standard American Chinese dish that incorporates crisp chicken, spice, and a tinge of orange flavoring. This recipe is derived from a dish a college roommate of mine used to make. If you guessed his name is David, then you would be correct. As with many of the other lunch dishes, this one is also great when served cold. This dish is a complete meal and doubles as a fantastic dinner that is quick to make.

Ready in 25 Minutes

15 minutes to prep and 10 minutes to cook

Ingredients (serves 4):

2 large chicken breasts

1 orange, cut and peeled

1 teaspoon of corn starch

4 teaspoon of vegetable oil

1 bag of precut broccoli florets (should equal roughly 2 cups)

1 tablespoon of minced ginger

¼ cup water (to mix with soy sauce)

3 tablespoons of soy sauce

¼ cup of orange juice

½ cup of chicken or vegetable broth

½ cup water (for help in cooking broccoli)

Step 1:

Take the chicken breasts and cut into long strips. Add the soy sauce to the ¼ cup of water and mix, set aside. During this step, make sure that your other ingredients are all set and ready to go. Once the pan heats up the cooking processes is very fast.

Step 2:

Add the vegetable oil to a large skillet warm over medium heat. Add the chicken strips and cook halfway – add the ginger and continue to cook the chicken until it is entirely done. Take the chicken and ginger out of the skillet and set aside.

Step 3:

Return to the skillet and add the broccoli. You should not need to add any additional oil but if when removing the chicken the pan was left dry, add an additional teaspoon. As the broccoli starts to lightly brown add the ½ cup of water and cover the skillet. Let the broccoli steam for 3 minutes. Check the broccoli to make sure that it is cooked through and not too raw.

Step 4:

Add the cooked chicken and ginger to the skillet. Add the soy sauce mixed with water, the orange juice, and the chicken broth. Mix these ingredients well and allow to cook for an additional 5 minutes. If the chicken or broccoli is beginning to be overcooked, change the heat to low or turn off the burner.

Step 5:

Add in the cornstarch and continue to mix. Once the cornstarch has been mixed in, add the orange peels to the top of the dish and cook for an additional minute or two. Serve right away.

DINNER RECIPES FOR THE HEALTHY BODY

Lightning Fast Curry Noodles – 3 SmartPoints Per Serving

This is a recipe I commonly refer to when I'm looking to make a quick dinner with just a bit of Asian flair. My favorite aspect to this recipe is that by using rice noodles you do not need to cook the noodles in a pot of boiling water. It can be made with just about any protein, including eggs or tofu. This particular version is vegetarian free, but adding cooked chicken or beef works just as well. This is my own recipe is supposed to mimic Singapore Noodles, a dish commonly found at Chinese restaurants throughout the country.

Ready In 20 Minutes:

10 minutes to prepare and 10 minutes to cook

Ingredients (serves 4)

3 large eggs

2 tablespoons whole milk (or half and half)

3 teaspoons of curry powder

2 tablespoons of vegetable oil

2 whole white mushrooms

1 bell pepper

1 package of Rice Noodles (you will want to go for medium thickness in the noodle – the particular brand does not matter)

2 tablespoons of soy sauce (low sodium soy sauce will *taste* more salty than regular soy sauce. If using low sodium soy then only use 1 tablespoon)

Step 1:

Take a large bowl or pot and fill it with warm water. The water does not need to approach boiling, and running hot water from your tap will suffice. Once the bowl is full, put the package of rice noodles into the water. You want to check back in a few minutes to make sure that every noodle is submerged in the water.

Step 2:

Slice the mushrooms and bell peppers into small slices. This dish will look a lot like a noodle stir fry, so cut the peppers in long strips and the mushrooms into thin slices.

Step 3:

While the noodles are soaking, use a small frying pan and with the milk and 3 eggs, make scrambled eggs. Once the eggs are made put them aside on a separate plate and cut the scrambled eggs into small pieces.

Step 4:

As the eggs are cooking, take a pan suitable for stir fry and add the vegetable oil. If you do not have a suitable stir fry pan, you can also use a standard pot for boiling pasta. Bring the heat to medium high and once the oil is hot add the mushrooms. As the mushrooms start to cook, add the peppers.

Step 5:

Strain the rice and noodles and add them to the pan with the mushrooms and the bell peppers. Note that the noodles should still appear to be a little bit brittle, do not worry as they will continue to cook in the pan.

Step 6:

As the noodles are cooking in the pan, add the soy sauce and mix thoroughly. Once the sauce is mixed, add the curry powder and stir thoroughly. The noodles should start to take on a dark yellowish color and at this point they should be thoroughly cooked through.

Step 7:

Add the cooked eggs to the pan, and then serve immediately. If the scrambled eggs are slightly cold, they will be warmed up through the cooked noodles.

Step 8:

Serve immediately and enjoy! This meal also works great for lunch. If you are unable to reheat the noodles while at work, they taste great just at room temperature.

Simple Season Chicken– 3 SmartPoints Per Serving

This recipe is a great healthy way to make seasoned chicken cutlets. These cutlets have just the right amount of seasoning and come packed with all the healthy protein of lean chicken breast. This recipe can altered slightly to make a lean type of chicken parmesan. See the altered steps 4 and 5 if you wish to go this route, otherwise this recipe is great with a side of spinach or any other side vegetable.

Ready In 35 Minutes

10 minutes to prepare and 25 minutes to cook

Ingredients (serves 4)

Chicken breast (use roughly 1 pound and cut into 4 large filets)

1/8 teaspoon paprika

¼ cup of parmesan cheese (grated finely)

½ teaspoon of garlic powder

1 teaspoon of parsley (optional)

black pepper to taste

3 tablespoons of dried breadcrumbs

Directions:

Step 1:

Preheat your oven to 400 degrees F or 205 degrees C

Step 2:

Take a small mixing bowl and add the breadcrumbs, grated parmesan, garlic powder, and paprika. Add a pinch of black pepper but know that you can add more while the chicken is cooking.

Step 3:

Take your sliced pieces of chicken breast and dip them into the bowl. Coat both sides of each piece of chicken. Since we are using a healthier version of traditional chicken parmesan, you might have some difficult having the mix stick to the chicken. It is best dip the chicken in the bowl right after you wash the chicken, using the moisture to get it to stick properly.

Step 4:

Prepare a nonstick baking tray and align the pieces of chicken towards the center of the baking tray.

Alternate for Chicken Parmesan: Using the Homemade Multi-Purpose Marina sauce (the next recipe in the book), lather the chicken liberally in 2-3 cups of sauce. You will need to use a deeper baking dish to cook the Chicken Parmesan. Once the sauce and chicken has been laid out, coat with shredded Parmesan Cheese and whole slices of mozzarella. To use an appropriate amount of cheese, only layer the cheese on top of the chicken filets. Note that this adds roughly 2 Smart Points to each serving.

Step 5:

Let the chicken bake in the oven for 25 minutes. Check at about 20 minutes as thinner pieces of chicken will cook more quickly. 25 minutes is around the upper limit for how long it will take to cook the chicken.

Alternate for Chicken Parmesan: Using the oven set to 400 degrees F, bake for 35-40 minutes.

Step 6: Remove the chicken form the baking tray and serve within 5-10 minutes.

Homemade Multi-Purpose Marinara – 3 Smart Points Per Serving

This is a great recipe to try out on the weekend and use all week long. Whether it's topping for Chicken Parmesan, dipping sauce for bread, or the foundation of a great pasta dish, this marinara sauce will leave you with plenty of options for how to enjoy it.

Ready in 30 Minutes

10 minutes to prepare and 20 minutes to cook

Ingredients (makes 1 quart)

2 large cloves of garlic

4 large tomatoes

1 28 ounce can of peeled tomatoes

3 tablespoons of olive oil (use extra virgin olive oil – the taste will make a huge difference)

1 ½ tablespoons of sugar

½ teaspoon of ground black pepper

1 teaspoon of salt

½ large white onion

Step 1:

Take your fresh tomatoes and dice them into small chunks. You can also optionally peel the skin from the tomatoes for a smoother sauce. During this step also chop your half onion and your garlic cloves.

Step 2:

In large sauce pan, heat the olive oil under a medium heat, add the diced onion. Wait until the onion is firmly sautéing before adding the garlic.

Step 3:

Add your chopped tomatoes and your can of tomatoes. Also stir in your black pepper and salt. Bring the heat up to medium high and wait for the sauce to boil. Stir frequently and let the sauce boil for 15 minutes.

Step 4:

Turn the heat down to low on the burner and let the sauce simmer for an additional 30 minutes.

Savory Grilled Salmon – 4 Smart Points Per Serving

If there's a common theme with this cookbook, it's the idea that healthy proteins are the foundation to a great diet. Even if you do not normally love salmon, or if you've never tried it, this recipe is certainly worth a shot. At 4 SmartPoints per serving, a side dish of potatoes and spinach will bring the total meal to a reasonable 6-7 SmartPoints, meanwhile the salmon will keep you full until morning.

Ready in 50 Minutes

30 minutes to prep and 20 minutes to cook

Ingredients (serves 4):

1 pound of skinless salmon fillet. You will want the thickness of the salmon to be about 1 inch.

¼ cup of soy sauce

Non-stick cooking spray

1 tablespoon of rice wine vinegar

¼ cup of dry sherry

1 tablespoon of brown sugar

1 teaspoon of garlic powder

1/8 teaspoon of ginger

Black pepper to taste

Step 1:

Preheat the oven to 375 degrees F or 190 degrees C. Make sure the grill rack is in the center of the oven.

Step 2:

Combine the sherry, soy sauce, brown sugar, vinegar, garlic powder, and ginger in a mixing bowl.

Step 3:

Dip the filets of salmon in the mixing bowl and place in the refrigerator for 20 minutes to marinade.

Step 4:

Place the remaining marinade in a small saucepan and heat on low. The marinade will begin to thicken as the salmon marinades in the refrigerator.

Step 5:

Spray the grill rack with non-stick spray and place the salmon filets on the rack. The cooking time for the salmon will differ greatly depending on thickness. As a guideline each side will need 4 to 8 minutes to cook through. The sign that the salmon is fully cooked is when it begins to flake.

Step 6:

Remove the salmon from the oven and place it on a large serving plate. Coat the salmon in the remaining marinade. Serve immediately.

Cheesy Baked Chicken – 5 SmartPoints Per Serving

I love this dish if for no other reason than it remind me that dieting does not need to omit cream and cheese. This chicken dish has all the flavor of a delicious casserole without any of the guilt. A simple side dish like a lightly tossed salad goes great, just be sure not to overdo it with the dressing.

Ready in 55 minutes:

10 minutes to prep and 45 minutes to cook

Ingredients (serves 8):

2 cups of cooked macaroni noodles

2 cups of 1% fat skin milk

2 cups of chopped boneless chicken breasts cut into cubes

8 ounces of low-fat shredded cheddar cheese

2 cups of undiluted cream of mushroom soup (I personally use Campbell's brand)

Step 1:

Preheat the oven to 350 degrees F or 175 degrees C.

Step 2:

Use a baking dish that is 2 inches deep, similar to a casserole dish, and place the cream of mushroom soup, the skim milk, cooked macaroni, shredded cheese, and uncooked chicken breasts into the baking tray. Mix thoroughly.

Step 3:

Place the baking tray in the center oven rack and bake for 35 minutes. At 35 minutes, take the baking tray out of the oven and remove a piece of chicken. Cut the chicken in half to see if it is cooked all the way through. Typically this recipe calls for 45 minutes, but if the chicken pieces are small enough the dish could be done in 35. Cook for an additional 10 minutes if needed.

Step 4:

45 minutes is the upper limit for cooking the casserole, but always make sure to slice the chicken and make sure that it is cooked all the way through. Small variables could mean cooking for an additional 5-10 minutes.

Step 5:

Let the dish cook for 10 minutes before serving.

Lean Mean Pork Chops – 3 SmartPoints Per Serving

In this recipe we are using our oven to bypass the unnecessary oil we'd get in by using a frying pan. This will lead to a more brazen pork that should be more tender. This dish takes longer than several of our other dinners and so use this time to experiment with side dishes. A vegetable melody goes great as the extra time gives you the opportunity to wash and cut your vegetables. You can also use the already heated oven for simple sliced baked potatoes – even the spices from the pork can be reused if you wish.

Ready in 70 Minutes

20 minutes to prep and 50 minutes to cook

Ingredients Needed (serves 4):

Non-stick cooking spray

1 large egg white

¼ teaspoon of ground ginger

1/8 teaspoon of garlic powder

2 tablespoon of pineapple juice

6 ounces of pork loin (try and get lean pork if available)

1 tablespoon of soy sauce

¼ teaspoon of paprika

1/3 cup dried breadcrumbs

¼ teaspoon of dried Italian seasoning

Step 1:

Preheat the oven to 350 degrees F or 175 degrees C

Step 2:

If you were able to purchase lean pork loin then you do not need to follow this step. If you were not able to purchase lean pork loin, trim away as much fat as you can. Do not worry about the taste – our seasoning will make up for the flavor.

Step 3:

In large mixing bowl, add the soy sauce, garlic powder, egg white, ginger, and pineapple juice. Mix well as the egg white is sometimes difficult to mix thoroughly.

Step 4:

Using a separate bowl, mix breadcrumbs, Italian seasoning, and the paprika.

Step 5:

Take the pork chops and dip them into the wet mixing bowl and then dip them into the dry mixing bowl. Coat the pork chops well but know that some ingredients will be left.

Step 6:

Lay the pork chops on the baking tray. Bake for 25-30 minutes on each side. Wait 3-5 minutes before serving.

Fast Cooking Scallops – 3 SmartPoints Per Serving

The hardest part of this recipe is the trip to the supermarket to purchase scallops. Do not fear as frozen scallops will work just fine, and if you are inexperienced cooking fish you also do not have to worry – this recipe is built upon the idea that perhaps this is your first time cooking fish in a pan. If you are unsure about whether to try this recipe, think about scallops as the 'meatier' shrimp. For a side dish, I recommend a baked potato and spinach or zucchini. The lemon goes great with subtle side dishes like these.

Ready in 20 Minutes

10 minutes to prep and 10 minutes to cook

Ingredients (serves 4):

1 pound of sea scallops, dried

2 tablespoons of all purpose flour

1 tablespoon of virgin olive oil

1 tablespoon of lemon juice

1 minced scallions

¼ teaspoon of salt

2 tablespoons of parsley

Pinch of sage (nice flavor, but not necessary if you don't already have this spice)

Step 1:

Take a mixing bowl and add the flour, scallions, and salt.

Step 2:

Take the scallops and dip them in the mixing bowl. Don't worry about how much of the mix ends up on the scallions – it should only be a small layer and does not necessary need to cover the scallops entirely.

Step 3:

Take a large skillet and heat the olive oil under medium heat. Toss the scallops one at a time into the pan. The scallops should could in about 4 minutes. Be careful not to overcook the scallops as they will become very though. You will know the scallops are done when they become impossible to see through the skin.

Step 4:

If the scallops were made in batches, add all of the scallops back into the pan, turning off the heat before you do so. Add the chopped parsley and lemon juice. Mix well and serve right away

9 789814 952019